SURGEON'S SURVIVAL GUIDE TO THE FOUNDATION YEARS

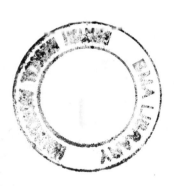
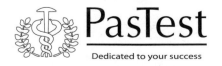

PasTest

Dedicated to your success

SURGEON'S SURVIVAL GUIDE TO THE FOUNDATION YEARS

by

Jonathan Ghosh MB BCh MD MRCS

Specialist Registrar in General/Vascular Surgery
Manchester
UK

and

Michael O Murphy BA MB BCh BAO MA MD MRCP
MRCS

Cardiac Surgery Fellow
Massachusetts General Hospital
Boston
USA

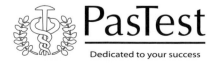
Dedicated to your success

© 2006 PASTEST LTD
Egerton Court
Parkgate Estate
Knutsford
Cheshire
WA16 8DX

Telephone: 01565 752000

First published 2006

ISBN: 1 904 627 846
       978 1904627845

A catalogue record for this book is available from the British Library.

The information contained within this book was obtained by the author from
reliable sources. However, while every effort has been made to ensure its
accuracy, no responsibility for loss, damage or injury occasioned to any person
acting or refraining from action as a result of information contained herein can
be accepted by the publishers or author.

PasTest Revision Books and Intensive Courses

PasTest has been established in the field of postgraduate medical education
since 1972, providing revision books and intensive study courses for doctors
preparing for their professional examinations.

Books and courses are available for the following specialties:

**MRCGP, MRCP Parts 1 and 2, MRCPCH Parts 1 and 2, MRCPsych, MRCS,
MRCOG Parts 1 and 2, DRCOG, DCH, FRCA, PLAB Parts 1 and 2.**

For further details contact:

PasTest, Freepost, Knutsford, Cheshire WA16 7BR
Tel: 01565 752000   Fax: 01565 650264
www.pastest.co.uk   enquiries@pastest.co.uk

Text prepared by Type Study, Scarborough, North Yorkshire
Printed and bound in the UK by Cambridge University Press, Cambridge

DEDICATION

To my family and friends for their unending patience and generosity.
MM

For Rosie and Jamie.
JG

We would both like to thank our surgical mentors past, present and future.

CONTENTS

PREFACE

An important change in NHS clinical practice that has arisen from *Modernising Medical Careers* is the introduction of the foundation programmes. During the first 2 years of professional practice, junior doctors are exposed to a broader variety of specialties in both the elective and emergency setting.

Although new graduates will have grounding in the principles of surgery in general, and the basic sciences, most will feel apprehensive about starting on a surgical firm and cross-covering other unfamiliar specialties, particularly at night. Most face the difficulty of providing the first port of call for problems in specialties that they may never rotate through and almost invariably do not go on to higher surgical training in. This handbook has been written to provide practical guidance on some of the more common problems faced in the different sub-specialties. It is designed principally for new foundation doctors but will also be of benefit to medical students and those approaching the Membership of the Royal College of Surgeons (MRCS) examinations.

Much of this text has been prepared by trainees and consultants at Manchester Royal Infirmary, and so we acknowledge the use of departmental protocols. This is not designed to be an exhaustive review of each of the sub-specialties and is not a substitute for directed reading from established texts. In addition there are many local and regional policies on how to deal with particular problems and these should be followed assiduously. However, we hope that it will act as a valuable aide-memoire for day-to-day use. When dealing with most problems the basic advanced life support (ALS) and Advanced Trauma Life Support (ATLS) principles form the cornerstone of initial management, with additional areas covered in the individual chapters.

J Ghosh

M O Murphy

CONTRIBUTORS

Andrew Carter

Research Fellow
Manchester Royal Infirmary
Manchester
UK

Grainne Colgan

SpR in Orthopaedic Surgery
Tallaght Hospital
Dublin

Ken Dunn

Consultant Burns and Plastic Surgeon
Wythenshawe Hospital
Manchester
UK

Jonathan Ghosh

Specialist Registrar in General/Vascular Surgery
Manchester Royal Infirmary
Manchester
UK

James Greenwood

Specialist Registrar in Respiratory Medicine/ITU
University Hospital
Aintree, Liverpool
UK

Nadeem Khwaja

Specialist Registrar in Plastic Surgery
Sandwell General Hospital
West Bromich
UK

Sadie Khwaja

Specialist Registrar in ENT
Hope Hospital and Pendlebury Childrens' Hospital
Salford
UK

J P McElwain

Consultant Orthopaedic Surgeon
Tallaght Hospital
Dublin
Ireland

Kenneth E McLaughlin

Consultant Cardiothoracic Surgeon
Manchester Royal Infirmary
Manchester
UK

Mary Murphy

Consultant Neurosurgeon
Addenbrooke's Hospital
Cambridge
UK

Michael O Murphy

Cardiac Surgery Fellow
Massachusetts General Hospital
Boston
USA

Richard Napier-Hemy

Consultant Urologist
Manchester Royal Infirmary
Manchester
UK

Shak Saeed

Consultant ENT Surgeon
Manchester Royal Infirmary
Manchester
UK

Michael G Walker

Consultant Vascular Surgeon
Manchester Royal Infirmary
Manchester
UK

Angus J M Watson

Consultant Colorectal Surgeon
Manchester Royal Infirmary
Manchester
UK

ABBREVIATIONS USED IN THIS BOOK

A&E	Accident and Emergency
AAA	abdominal aortic aneurysm
ABG	arterial blood gases
ABPI	ankle–brachial pressure index
ACE	angiotensin-converting enzyme
ACL	anterior cruciate ligament
AFP	α-feto protein
ALT	alanine aminotransferase
AP	anteroposterior
APTT	activated partial thromboplastin time
ARDS	acute respiratory distress syndrome
ARF	acute renal failure
ASIS	anterior superior iliac spine
AST	aspartate aminotransferase
ATLS	Advanced Trauma Life Support
AXR	abdominal X-ray
bd	twice daily
BM	blood glucose
BMI	body mass index
BP	blood pressure
BPH	benign prostatic hyperplasia
CABG	coronary artery bypass graft
CEA	carcinoembryonic antigen
CMV	continuous mandatory ventilation
CPAP	continuous positive airways pressure
CRP	C-reactive protein
CSDH	chronic subdural haematoma
CT	computed tomography
CVP	central venous pressure
CXR	chest X-ray
DIC	disseminated intravascular coagulation
DVT	deep vein thrombosis
EAM	external auditory meatus
ECG	electrocardiogram
ELISA	enzyme-linked immunosorbent assay
ENT	ear, nose and throat
ERCP	endoscopic retrograde cholangiopancreatography
ESR	erythrocyte sedimentation rate

EVAR	endovascular aneurysm repair
FBC	full blood count
FFP	fresh frozen plasma
FNA	fine needle aspiration
FTSG	full thickness skin graft
GA	general anaesthetic
GFR	glomerular filtration rate
GGT	γ-glutamyl transferase
GKI	glucose-potassium-insulin
GP	general practitioner
GTN	glyceryl trinitrate
Hb	Haemoglobin
hCG	β-human chorionic gonadotrophin
HRT	hormone replacement therapy
im	intramuscular
INR	international normalised ratio
IPPV	intermittent positive pressure ventilation
ITU	intensive therapy unit
iv	intravenous
IVU	intravenous urogram
KUB	kidney-ureter-bladder
LDH	lactate dehydrogenase
LFT	liver function test
LMWH	low-molecular-weight heparin
MAP	mean arterial pressure
MEN	multiple endocrine neoplasia
MI	myocardial infarction
MSU	mid-stream urine
NAI	non-accidental injury
NIV	non-invasive ventilation
NSAID	non-steroidal anti-inflammatory drug
OCP	oral contraceptive pill
ORIF	open reduction and internal fixation
PCA	patient-controlled analgesia
PCI	percutaneous intervention
PCR	polymerase chain reaction
PE	pulmonary embolism
PEEP	positive end-expiratory pressure
PEG	percutaneous endoscopic gastrostomy
PET	positron emission tomography
PID	pelvic inflammatory disease

PPI	proton pump inhibitor
PSA	prostate-specific antigen
PTA	percutaneous transluminal angioplasty
PTC	percutaneous trans-hepatic cholangiography
RICE	rest, ice, compression and elevation
RRT	renal replacement therapy
SAH	subarachnoid haemorrhage
sc	subcutaneous
SIMV	synchronised intermittent mandatory ventilation
SIRS	systemic inflammatory response syndrome
SSG	split thickness skin graft
STD	sexually transmitted disease
TDR	targeted diabetic regimen
tds	three times daily
TFT	thyroid function test
TIA	transient ischaemic attack
TNF	tumour necrosis factor
TPN	total parenteral nutrition
TRUS	transrectal ultrasound
TSH	thyroid stimulating hormone
TWOC	trial without catheter
U&E	urea and electrolytes
USS	ultrasound scan
UTI	urinary tract infection
VATS	video-assisted thoracic surgery
WCC	white cell count

CHAPTER 1

THE BASICS

J GHOSH AND M O MURPHY

Surgical placements can be among the most educational and enjoyable of your rotation. Generally, you will get out as much as you put in. The following guidelines, applicable to all foundation placements, will help you get the most out of your time on a surgical firm:

- **Be mindful of your limitations and do not be afraid to ask for help**. Senior doctors, predecessors and nurses are all sources of advice. All of them were once new to the post and they all know what it is like to start at the deep end. No one expects you to know it all straight after medical school. Asking for help is how everybody learns and there is no such thing as a stupid question. Happily, most ward tasks will rapidly become routine. However, repetition of mistakes during the early stages of the job, or not understanding why you are doing a particular task will escalate and lead to problems later on. Taking on too much, guesswork and ignorance of your job requirements will lead to errors and repercussions.

- **Look after yourself**. Eat well and take rests. You will not do service to your patients, your team or yourself if you are run down. If you feel stressed – stop and ask yourself why? Diagnosing stress and its cause is the first step to alleviating it. If you feel lost, speak to your superior or educational supervisor. If you feel over-worked, remember there is support available. Most people are happy to help out. Do *not* suffer in silence.

- **Be organised, anticipate and prioritise**. Each day, many demands will be made of you and it will feel like you are needed in three places at once. The only way to survive is to prioritise jobs and do the urgent ones first. This is not always simple, particularly at the start of the job, but it does become easier with experience. Before the morning ward round, make sure that you have an up-to-date patient list and have printouts of the results of recent blood and other investigations with you, so that ill patients can be recognised as you go around. During the ward round jot down all required tasks on your patient list. Carry a clipboard, note pad or PDA for this purpose. Do not rely on memory alone – you will forget things. After the ward round, take 5 minutes to review your job list and decide what needs to done as a priority and what can wait until later. Prioritise according to how unwell the patient is and impending deadlines such as theatre. If there is more than one house officer on your team, learn to 'divide and conquer' by equally allocating jobs and responsibilities. Anticipating problems and tasks helps organisation. For example, make blood requests in advance. Try not to allow tasks to build up – clear the decks as soon and as often as you can. Such measures will improve efficiency and time management. If you are asked to take a blood test or request an X-ray, do not simply do so and then forget about it. Try to understand why it is needed (ask if you're not sure), check the results and act on them. This may merely mean informing your senior, but do not get into the habit of leaving tests until the next day before looking at the results. Early intervention saves lives.

- **Remember that you are now a professional**. So try to act like one. This requires that you are reliable, keep promises and be a team player. We all get tired, frustrated and annoyed. However, nothing is gained, and an awful lot is lost, if you release frustrations on nursing staff, patients and colleagues. Similarly it is poor form to openly criticise colleagues. Such behaviour will give you a bad reputation, which will be difficult to recover from.
- **Educational opportunities are everywhere**. Even if you have absolutely no intention of pursuing a career in surgery, there are core skills that will serve you well no matter what line you go into. Try to go to theatre whenever possible. In particular, day case 'lump and bumps' lists are a good opportunity to get some cutting experience. Try to fix some sessions with one of the registrars to learn suturing and hand tying. Volunteer to do as many practical procedures as possible.
- **Unwind**. Don't forget your life outside the ward. Book time off early. Keep in touch with old friends and also make an effort to socialise with colleagues (medical and non-medical). Getting to know colleagues outside the working environment makes day-to-day life a lot more relaxed and enjoyable.

Table 1.1 Some useful educational websites and organisations

Clinical	
SURGICAL-TUTOR	www.surgical-tutor.org.uk
EMedicine	www.emedicine.com
GPnotebook	www.gpnotebook.co.uk
PubMed	www.pubmed.com
British National Formulary	www.bnf.org/bnf/
National Electronic Library for Health	www.nelh.nhs.uk/
Careers	
Royal Colleges of Surgery	www.rcsed.ac.uk
	www.rcseng.ac.uk
	www.rcpsg.ac.uk
	www.rcsi.ie
Association of Surgeons in Training (ASiT)	www.asit.org
General Medical Council (GMC)	www.gmc-uk.org
GMC's good medical practice	www.gmc-uk.org/guidance/good_medical_practice/index.asp
British Medical Association (BMA)	www.bma.org.uk
Modernising Medical Careers	www.mmc.nhs.uk/pages/foundation
Advice/support	
BMA counselling service	www.bma.org.uk/doctorsfordoctors Tel: 020 7383 6739
Doctors' Support Network	www.dsn.org.uk
Sick Doctors Trust	www.sick-doctors-trust.co.uk

Table 1.1 *Continued*

Protection societies	
Medical Defence Union	www.the-mdu.com Tel: 0800 716 646
Medical Protection Society	www.medicalprotection.org Tel: 0845 605 4000
Medical and Dental Defence Union of Scotland	www.mddus.com Tel: 0141 221 5858

DOCUMENTATION AND COMMUNICATION

Documentation in the patient's notes by medical staff – both junior and senior – has always been notoriously poor. In contemporary healthcare this is unacceptable, as the medico-legal significance of clinical notes cannot be overstated:

> If it hasn't been documented (or is illegible) then it hasn't been done!

Clear, easily decipherable notes remain the most important mode of information transfer between healthcare professionals and are essential for efficient patient management.

It is often the foundation doctor who is left to write in the notes during wards rounds – which are more often than not rushed. If there is any doubt about what has been said, then do not be shy about asking for clarification so that you record the correct information. Try to write in the notes as you go around, rather than retrospectively, as it is easy to forget important information. Patients now have the right to full access to their medical notes – bear this in mind when writing information about them and keep written information professional. Good documentation is the first step in getting yourself a good reputation.

The following points should be adhered to:

- Make sure the correct patient's name is written on all history sheets
- Keep handwriting legible. Note-form annotation is perfectly fine providing it conforms to commonly used formats. Use black ink
- Date and time all entries
- If on a ward round, document who is leading it and their designation

- Document current patient status, observation findings, investigation findings and plan. In this way, a third party can easily work out the status of the patient and how they are being treated. (See also Postoperative monitoring, page 22)
- When documenting a conversation with a patient, also record who else was present. Similarly, if a chaperoned examination has been performed, note down who was with you
- If documenting a clerking, adhere to the scheme: presenting complaint/history of presenting complaint/past medical history/drug history/allergy/social history/review of systems/examination. Do not forget to document age and occupation and your differential diagnosis
- At the end, sign and print your name and designation along with your bleep number

TAKE-HOME PRESCRIPTIONS

Take-home prescriptions are one of many repetitive tasks that you will have to perform. However, this is not to say that it is not important. 'Take homes' serve two purposes. The first is to provide the patient with medication and the second is to give the general practitioner (GP) a brief summary of the patient's hospital stay. Put yourself in the position of the pharmacist or GP. A few seconds extra will make life easier for everyone and stop angry phone calls from pharmacists who cannot read your handwriting.

X-RAY REQUESTS

Similarly as above, investigation requests – particular radiological – need to be written clearly and concisely. Remember that the request will be to a consultant or other senior ranked doctor, who will be relying on your disclosure of clinical details on which to base their interpretation.

Sending fully completed requests is a good way of establishing good relations with a radiologist. This will become very useful during your placements.

REFERRALS

You will be regularly asked to make a referral to another specialty. Whether this is done verbally or in writing, the principles are the same. First and foremost, understand why you are making a referral and what you want it to achieve. Spend 5 minutes familiarising yourself with the case, relevant history and investigation results. If it is a verbal referral, have these details to hand before you make the phone call. When facing a consultant or middle-grade doctor, you will make a good impression (and develop a good reputation) if you can demonstrate that you are thinking ahead. Conversely, it looks sloppy if you cannot convey the correct or relevant information and any questions are answered by a 'don't know'.

Before writing or telephoning your referral, it is useful to go through the wording in your own head before committing to it. What you want is a short and 'to the point' referral with relevant information and no 'waffling'. As you gain experience, this will become natural, but it does take practice. Remember to be polite: request – don't demand.

THE OPERATING THEATRE

A theatre complex will consist of a number of individual operating theatres. There is usually a main reception where patients and visitors are checked in, a common room, changing rooms and a recovery area where patients go after surgery to be stabilised before return to the ward. You will have to change into theatre scrubs and a cap prior to entering the inner theatre suite to reduce transmission of pathogens. It is unacceptable to leave theatre without changing out of scrubs or without a covering garment. Theatre caps and masks should be worn inside the operating theatre. Some orthopaedic theatres will have an inner 'tent' as a further level of infection control.

The operating room is deceptively complex. The typical operating theatre will have an anaesthetic room, a scrubbing-up room where the surgeons and scrub staff will scrub and gown up, a sluice and the main operating area. To reduce atmospheric contaminations it generates a positive pressure to push air and aerosol contaminates away from theatre and the operative field. A standard theatre will perform 20 air changes per hour, although orthopaedic theatres can achieve several hundred air changes per hour. It is for this reason that theatre doors need to stay closed.

A sister/charge nurse co-ordinates staff and the smooth operational running of the theatre list. A gowned scrub nurse will be present during the surgery to provide the operating surgeon with instruments as requested. There is usually a 'runner' to get sutures and extra items. Assisting the anaesthetist is an operating departmental assistant. The theatre suite will have its own porters to transfer patients to and from theatre. Increasingly, nursing staff with higher training are taking a more involved role in operations. Surgical care practitioners work both inside and outside the operating room and can perform interventions under direct, indirect or proximal supervision. Advance scrub practitioners do not perform surgery but can provide assistance.

Before surgery, usually the day before, a theatre list is circulated to individual wards stating the running order for the day's list. If you are interested in seeing or assisting in a particular operation, this will give an indication when it will be. If you plan to go to theatre to watch some cases, spend a short time reading about the operation. You will profit a lot more if know the basics – and the operating surgeon will probably talk through the case more if you show that you are keen!

Use any opportunity to learn how to tie surgical knots, learn instrument names and learn about different operations.

If you are not scrubbed in theatre

- Make sure that you are wearing a cap and correct footwear
- Do not touch or come into close proximity to any sterile draped area
- Be careful when moving lights – do not touch sterile handles
- Check with the surgeon or nursing staff from where it is best to observe the operation. A stand is usually available to improve the view

If you are scrubbed in theatre

- Keep you hands close to your chest or on a draped area to avoid desterilisation
- Check that light handles are sterile before touching them
- If you feel faint or light-headed, tell the surgeon or nurse and step back from the operating table immediately. Find somewhere to sit down, and if necessary descrub to get a drink and a snack
- If you get a needle stick injury, follow the hospital occupational health protocol. There are no exceptions to this

- If you accidentally desterilise your glove, tell the nursing staff immediately and they will get you a replacement. If you contaminate your gown, re-scrub straight away

EMERGENCY LISTS

All hospitals will run a dedicated theatre to deal with trauma and emergency cases. These patients are usually managed by the on-call team but it is often the foundation doctor who has to book them: emergency patients have to be 'booked' (there is usually a booking sheet that needs to be filled) and the on-call anaesthetist and theatre staff informed. Most orthopaedic units will in addition have a trauma co-ordinator who facilitates the smooth running of the emergency theatre and is the usual first point of contact provided that the patient can wait until the next list. When you start your post, make sure that you are familiar with the theatre booking procedure. Before you book a patient, you will almost certainly need to know the following:

- The patient's name, date of birth and hospital number
- Ward
- Operation, and side
- Who will be doing the operation
- An idea of the patient's history and investigation results, the anaesthetist will want to know
- When the patient last had food/drink
- If the patient has methicillin-resistant *Staphylococcus aureus* (MRSA); theatre staff will need to make special arrangements

SCRUBBING-UP

Maintenance of sterilisation in theatre is vital in reducing the morbidity and mortality associated with postoperative infections. Of paramount importance is a sound scrubbing-up technique. There is no substitute to getting a scrub nurse or sister to demonstrate the correct procedure. Scrubbing-up involves washing, gowning and gloving.

PREPARATION FOR SCRUBBING

Do not leave valuable objects unattended in the changing room – keep them in a locker or on your person. Remove your watch and place your bleep to one side. It is irritating to have your bleep persistently going off under your surgical gown where nobody can attend to it.

Make sure you are in the correct theatre scrubs and shoes, are wearing a theatre cap and have a mask. Put on a visor and a waterproof plastic gown under the sterile operating gown if a messy operation is anticipated. In addition 'double glove' if there is a perceived significant risk of viral transmission. Learn in advance what glove size you are. Open a gown and lay it out on the scrub table. Drop gloves onto the gown without directly touching it.

WASHING

Adjust the elbow taps to deliver water at a comfortable temperature. Wet your hands, apply cleaning detergent, and work up a good lather. Rub hands, then forearms to above the elbows for one complete minute. Wash your forearms. Repeat three times and then rinse the suds from your hands while keeping your hands higher than your elbows. Turn off the taps with your elbows. Dry your hands first, then the forearms, with a sterile towel. Try not to bring a wet (unsterile) towel back to a dry area.

GOWNING

Hold the gown away from your body, high enough to be well above the floor. Allow it to drop open, and put your arms into the arm holes. Theatre staff will tie your gown from behind and assist you with the waist strap.

GLOVING

Be careful to touch only the inner surface of the gloves. Grasp the palmar aspect of the turned down cuff of a glove, and pull it on to your opposite hand. Leave its cuff for the moment. Put the fingers of your already gloved hand under the inverted cuff of the other glove, and pull it on to your bare hand. If a glove becomes torn or inadvertently contaminated, remove it by grasping its cuff from the outside, and pull it down over your palm. Give a few seconds for your hand to dry before putting a fresh glove on as above. Once gowned and gloved, walk with your hands above waist level. Do not touch undraped, non-sterile surfaces and be careful with light handles. Do not place your hands in the operative field unnecessarily.

PREOPERATIVE ASSESSMENT FOR ELECTIVE SURGERY

PRINCIPLES OF ELECTIVE PREOPERATIVE ASSESSMENT

The aim of preoperative assessment is to identify the patient's co-morbidities that may affect surgery and may adversely affect postoperative recovery. Careful evaluation of the patient may uncover areas that require treatment or investigation. Occasionally evidence is found of undiagnosed disease or poor control of known pathology, resulting in a referral to an appropriate specialist. Increasingly this is carried out in co-operation with anaesthetists.

The National Institute for Health and Clinical Excellence (NICE; www.nice.org.uk) has issued guidance on preoperative investigations, which are determined by patient age and the American Society of Anesthesiologists (ASA) grade (see Table 1.2). Furthermore, most surgical departments will have protocols for preoperative evaluation and work-up for elective patients. Make sure that you have access to these and are familiar with them. Mistakes can have grave consequences or lead to cancellations.

The following sections provide an outline of elective preoperative assessment.

History

- Symptoms/condition requiring surgery
- History of presenting illness including summary of relevant investigations
- Past medical history and medication. Note usage of steroids, anticoagulants, antiplatelets and diabetic medication
- Note any allergies – particularly antibiotics
- Review of systems. Of relevance to preoperative patients are cardiac and respiratory systems. Any symptoms suggestive of previous deep vein thrombosis (DVT)?
- Social history. How will the patient cope following discharge?

A number of risk prediction systems have been devised, but the most widespread and easiest is the ASA scoring system (Table 1.2) ('+E' is used as a suffix for emergency cases).

Table 1.2 ASA classification for preoperative assessment

ASA class	Definition	Mortality (%)
I	Healthy individual	0.05
II	Mild systemic disease with no limitation to daily activity	0.4
III	Severe systemic disease limiting daily activity but not incapacitating	4.5
IV	Incapacitating systemic illness which is constantly life-threatening	25
V	Not expected to survive 24 hours with or without surgery	50

Examination

All systems – focusing on presenting complaint, cardiac and respiratory examination.

Investigations

- Haemoglobin (Hb): all females, men over 60 years and anyone with cardiovascular symptoms or disease
- Urea and electrolytes (U&E): all diabetic patients, those with a renal history, those using medication that influence renal function (angiotensin-converting enzyme (ACE) inhibitors, diuretics, steroids) and anyone over 60 years
- Electrocardiogram (ECG): if over 40 years (men), 50 years (women) or history of diabetes or heart disease
- Chest X-ray (CXR): if cardiac/respiratory history, undergoing thoracic or upper abdominal surgery, or if a malignancy is present
- Echocardiogram and pulmonary function tests: for major surgery as directed by local hospital guidelines

PREPARATION

- Check results of investigations
- Crossmatch if major surgery intended as per hospital protocol
- Consent to be taken by senior member of surgical team as per Department of Health guidelines (below)

ON ADMISSION

- Nil by mouth for 6 hours preoperatively. Intravenous (iv) rehydration during this time. Be careful not to overload elderly people and those with cardiac failure with fluids. Liaise with senior staff if there is any doubt
- Prescribe bowel preparation as per hospital guidelines
- Full bowel clearance for colonoscopy, colonic surgery, rectal surgery
- Phosphate enema on morning of surgery – anal surgery, flexible sigmoidoscopy
- DVT prophylaxis – low-molecular-weight heparin (LMWH) and TED stockings
- Preoperative antibiotics as per hospital guideline
- Ensure that relevant X-rays or scans are available to go to theatre with the patient
- If the operation is unilateral, carefully mark the side with marker pen
- If a stoma is required, arrange for the stoma site to be marked, preferably by a specialist stoma therapist

CONSENT

The GMC states that the professional obtaining written consent for a procedure must have 'comprehensive understanding of the procedure or treatment, how it is carried out, and the risks attached to it'. Thus in practice, written consent can only be taken by a senior doctor or one who has completed a course as per Trust practice. Further guidance can be found at the Department of Health's website (www.dh.gov.uk/PolicyAndGuidance/HealthAndSocialCareTopics/Consent/).

SPECIAL PREOPERATIVE CONSIDERATIONS

RISKS OF MORTALITY FOLLOWING MYOCARDIAL INFARCTION

The timing of surgery following a myocardial infarction (MI) influences perioperative mortality as summarised in the box below.

RISK OF PERIOPERATIVE MORTALITY FOLLOWING SURGERY IN A PATIENT WITH HISTORY OF MI

- <3 weeks – 80%
- 3 weeks–3 months – 20–30%
- 3–6 months – 5–15%
- >6 months – 1–4%
- Perioperative MI mortality 50%

Baseline perioperative MI rate is 0.2% of which half are silent and most are on the third postoperative day

---

DIABETIC PATIENTS

All diabetic patients should receive their usual medication on the day before surgery. Patients with poorly controlled diabetes may need to be commenced on a sliding scale. Discuss with anaesthetist/surgeon and diabetology team if necessary. See also Table 1.3.

Table 1.3 Blood sugar management chart

	Type 1	Type 2	Non-diagnosed
Day before operation	Usual insulin	Usual tablets	Not applicable
Day of operation (am case)	No am insulin, start sliding scale in theatre	Usual tablets (check with anaesthetist)	Not applicable
Day of operation (pm case)	Usual am insulin plus light breakfast. Dextrose/saline infusion if BM < 3.0 mmol/l	Usual am tablets plus light breakfast. Dextrose/saline infusion 100 ml/h if BM < 3.0 mmol/l	Not applicable
In theatre	Commence on TDR scale	Commence on insulin if BM > 7.0 mmol/l	Commence on insulin if BM > 7.0 mmol/l
Day 1 after operation	Continue with iv sliding scale if not eating. Otherwise, stop iv sliding scale. Recommence usual sc insulin regimen plus commence 4-hourly sc sliding scale	Continue iv sliding scale if not eating. Otherwise, stop iv sliding scale plus commence on a 4-hourly sc sliding scale. Continue giving usual diabetic tablets	Continue iv sliding scale if not eating. Otherwise stop iv sliding scale. Commence on tablets if BM > 7 mmol/l. Metformin (± gliclazide) if overweight. Gliclazide if thin
Remainder of stay	Continue monitoring. BM should be back to normal control	Continue monitoring, control should be back to normal	Continue monitoring and fine tune medication

Preoperative management

Diabetic patients having surgery need close blood glucose (BM) control perioperatively. The anaesthetist will usually advise when this is to be started. This is usually achieved using a sliding scale insulin infusion or a glucose-potassium-insulin (GKI) protocol depending on local preference. Generally, this should be continued until the patient is eating and drinking normally in the postoperative period, at which point the patient's usual diabetic medication can be restarted. Ideally, all diabetic patients should be first on an operation list.

For patients first on the list:

- Type 1 diabetes – usual insulin will not be given and the patient is commenced on a sliding scale in theatre (preferably the targeted diabetic regimen (TDR))
- Type 2 – usual oral diabetic medication should be given unless the anaesthetist asks for it to be withheld

For patients second on the list:

- Type 1 – usual insulin will be given and the patient will be given a light breakfast. BM will be monitored hourly on the ward, and if it decreases to < 3.0 mmol/l a dextrose saline infusion will be commenced at 100 ml/h. The patient will be commenced on a sliding scale in theatre
- Type 2 – the patient will be given a light breakfast and the usual oral diabetic medication should be given unless the anaesthetist asks for it to be withheld

Postoperative management

Postoperatively, all patients must have hourly BM measurements until the glucose level stabilises. If BM is less than 3.0 mmol/l, patients should be commenced on a dextrose/saline infusion at 100 ml/h. The insulin infusion is continued and usual diabetic tablets are given. Most patients are able to discontinue the insulin infusion on the second postoperative day, or when eating.

Oral medication

Metformin

Metformin augments the sensitivity of the insulin receptor. It should not be discontinued and it should be given following surgery as soon as the patient can take oral medication. It is known to interact with intravenous/arterial contrast medium and should be avoided in patients undergoing angiography.

Gliclazide, glipizide, etc

These agents augment the insulin receptor sensitivity and promote the release of intrinsic insulin. In addition, they act on potassium channels to theoretically counteract the effect of agents such as nicorandil and may even promote the risk of ischaemia. This effect has not, however, been fully evaluated. These agents may need to be stopped on the day of operation.

Recommencing oral medication

All tablets should be given on the first postoperative day to control the blood sugar. The patient should remain on a dextrose/saline infusion until they are drinking adequately.

Patients on iv sliding scales

Patients should remain on an iv sliding scale for up to 48 hours, after which it can be stopped.

- Type 1 – usual insulin regimen should be recommenced
- Type 2 – continue usual tablets

Patients with previously undiagnosed diabetes

- If overweight (> 120% of ideal body weight): commence metformin 500 mg bd increasing to up to 1000 mg tds. Gliclazide 80 mg od or bd may also be given
- If not overweight: commence on gliclazide 80 mg od increasing to up to 160 mg bd

In addition all these patients must be prescribed a 4-hourly subcutaneous (sc) regimen (5 units if BM > 7.0 mmol/l; 10 units if BM > 10 mmol/l).

PATIENTS TAKING STEROIDS

Change to iv hydrocortisone to avoid adrenal shutdown, and recommence when eating normally. It is essential to appreciate that any patient on long-term steroids will have impaired adrenal function and is likely to cope badly with the stress of surgery when endogenous steroid production is increased. This means replacing oral steroids with iv steroids to avoid an addisonian crisis. See Table 1.4.

Table 1.4 Steroid equivalence

Hydrocortisone 20 mg	Triamcinalone 4 mg
Prednisolone 5 mg	Betamethasone 0.75 mg
Methylprednisolone 4 mg	Dexamethasone 0.75 mg

PATIENTS ON ANTICOAGULATION

- International normalised ratio (INR) should be < 1.5 for most operations, and 1 if a spinal/epidural is to be used
- Stop warfarin 3 days before surgery
- Intravenous heparin needed while off warfarin if patient has a prosthetic heart valve. Maintain activated partial thromboplastin time (APTT) ratio at 2–3

PATIENTS TAKING ANTIPLATELET MEDICATION (CLOPIDOGREL, ASPIRIN)

- Discuss with anaesthetist
- Stop 1 week prior to surgery
- In the emergency setting a platelet transfusion will reverse effects

WOMEN ON HORMONE REPLACEMENT THERAPY/ORAL CONTRACEPTIVE PILL

- Combined oral contraceptive pill (OCP) needs to be stopped 1 month before operation
- Progesterone-only OCP can be continued
- Hormone replacement therapy (HRT) needs DVT prophylaxis (LMWH)

SICKLE CELL DISEASE

Sickle cell disease is common in patients of Afro-Caribbean origin. This arises from an autosomal recessive single amino acid substitution (val → glu) on the haemoglobin β chain, which results in a less soluble molecule (HbS). Sickle cell anaemia occurs in homozygotes, whereas heterozygotes carry the sickle trait. Patients, especially homozygotes, require close monitoring as they are at high risk of sickling complication both intra- and postoperatively. Sickling complications include:

- Thrombotic crises – severe pain particularly in bones
- Aplastic crises – lethargy and pallor
- Sequestration – particularly in spleen and liver. Associated anaemia can become significant

Prevention of complications is the ideal. This requires liaison with the anaesthetist. The patient must be kept oxygenated and hydrated as sickling occurs when haemoglobin is deoxygenated. If sickle crisis is suspected, then senior help is needed. In the meantime:

- Patients often have chronic anaemia but transfusion may be required to maintain Hb of 90–100 g/l (9–10 g/dl)
- Maintain warmth
- Ensure adequate analgesia at all stages
- Opioid analgesia
- High-flow oxygen
- Intravenous access and rehydration
- Maintenance of warmth
- Crossmatch, full blood count (FBC), blood culture, CXR
- Broad-spectrum antibiotics, if pyrexial

PREOPERATIVE CHECKLIST

- Review of past medical history, drug history and allergies
- Consent
- Review blood results
- Group and save/crossmatch blood as per unit protocol
- X-rays/scans available
- Markings – side of surgery/stoma site
- Bowel preparation written up if required

- Intravenous maintenance fluids; beware of dehydration in elderly patients having bowel preparation
- Review any preoperative orders in notes or clinic letter, eg high-dependency unit (HDU)/intensive therapy unit (ITU)

DAY CASE SURGERY

A day case is a patient who is admitted for investigation or operation on a planned basis and returns home in less than 24 hours. Around half of all elective general surgical operations are performed as day cases, although it has been envisaged that this will increase to up to three-quarters. This is advantageous as waiting lists are reduced, costs are less, there is reduced demand for inpatient beds, reduced risk of cancellation, less risk of cross-infection and improved patient satisfaction.

Any operation or procedure can be performed as a day case, provided that it is of short duration, there is minimal bleeding and only basic postoperative analgesia is required. Both local and general anaesthetic cases can be undertaken as day cases.

Patients are discharged once orientated, mobile, comfortable and observationally stable. Contact details are provided in case of problems and outpatient follow-up arranged. Facilities must be available to arrange inpatient admission if needed following surgery, if there are any complications, concern regarding recovery and unexpected discomfort.

The key to a successful day case service is careful patient selection.

PATIENT CRITERIA FOR DAY CASE SURGERY

- Age < 70 years
- ASA 1 or 2
- BMI < 30 kg/m^2
- Availability of a responsible adult
- Access to a telephone
- Live within 1 hour from hospital

POSTOPERATIVE MONITORING

Patients require daily review, which must be documented in the case notes. The aim of the daily review is to guide and supervise recovery, to diagnose any complications and intervene early. The following checklist provides an outline of minimum requirements for postoperative review and documentation (although this should be individualised to the patient, surgery and supervising consultant).

- Note the number of days post-op
- Observations:

  - Pulse
  - Blood pressure
  - Temperature
  - Oxygen saturation
  - Urine output

- Drain/nasogastric tube output
- Check fluid input/output balance
- Pain control
- Chest auscultation
- Examination of wound and operative site
- Review for specific complications associated with surgery
- Review medication – including DVT prophylaxis, antibiotics, analgesia
- Review blood results/X-rays

  - Is transfusion required?
  - Potassium levels

- Review and prescribe fluid regimen based on U&E and fluid balance for past 24 hours
- Feeding/drinking/nutrition/bowel movement
- Mobility
- Note any abnormalities and an action plan for the next 24 hours

For details of specific postoperative complications see:

- Postoperative pyrexia – pages 24–26
- Wound infection – pages 25–27
- Respiratory distress/pneumonia – pages 355–356
- Chest pain – pages 360–362
- Renal failure – pages 366–368
- Arrhythmia – page 362
- Confusion – page 365

ENHANCED RECOVERY

Modern surgical management of postoperative patients is based on the philosophy of minimising inpatient postoperative care. Some of the old surgical dogma of bed rest, starvation, staged re-introduction of oral fluids and diet, and bowel preparation are now being challenged. Evidence-based approaches to postoperative care have led to a decreased requirement for prolonged stays. Foundation-year doctors are key in managing these advancements. When starting your placement, find out from senior colleagues the postoperative care practice followed for your consultant's patients.

SURGICAL WOUNDS

WOUND INFECTION

Surgical wounds may be classified as clean, clean-contaminated, contaminated and dirty. The rates of infection for these types of wound and the associated risk factors for infection are summarised in Tables 1.5 and 1.6, respectively.

History

Check the details of surgery and whether there was a pre-existing infection. Also enquire into pre-existing risk factors for infection (see Table 1.6). In particular, enquire about diabetes and preoperative steroid use and nutritional state.

The patient may complain of increasing pain from the wound. There may be a purulent discharge or area of erythema.

Table 1.5 Rates of infection associated with different wound types

Type of wound	Description	Infection rate (%)
Clean	Uninflamed tissue with no genitourinary/ gastrointestinal tract entry	< 2
Clean-contaminated	Entry to hollow viscus other than colon with minimal contamination	8–10
Contaminated	Spillage from hollow viscus, eg colon, operation fractures or bites	12–20
Dirty	Frank pus, perforated viscus, traumatic wound	> 25

Table 1.6 Factors leading to wound infection

Operative factors	Patient factors
Emergency surgery	Extremes of age
Extended preoperation admission	Poor nutritional status
Site of incision, eg perianal	Obesity
Excessive tension	Diabetes mellitus
Poor tissue handling	Alcoholism
Preoperation shaving	Immunosuppression
Necrotic tissue	Cardiac failure
Tissue ischaemia	Renal failure
Faecal peritonitis	Hepatic failure
Intra-abdominal abscess	Respiratory failure

Examination

- Look for redness, heat, swelling and tenderness
- There may be discharging pus
- Check for any fluctuant areas and whether the infection is superficial or deep and whether there is an underlying abscess
- Are the skin edges closed or distracted?

A serosanguineous discharge from a wound 1 week following abdominal surgery may suggest wound dehiscence (see below).

Treatment

Superficial cellulitis without an abscess can be observed if the patient is healthy, there is no systemic sepsis or pyrexia, the infection is localised and not expanding. Otherwise start antibiotics depending on the suspected causative organism. If there is pus, the wound will need to be opened and dressed appropriately.

WOUND DEHISCENCE

Wound dehiscence means all the layers of the wound are open, with exposed underlying viscera. It occurs typically 5–7 days postoperatively and **should be suspected if there is a serosanguineous discharge from the wound**. Abdominal wound dehiscence is associated with a mortality of 30% and must be dealt with emergently.

In the event of wound dehiscence, cover the wound with sterile saline or Betadine-soaked gauze, commence broad-spectrum antibiotics, keep the patient nil by mouth, start an iv infusion to maintain hydration and give opioid analgesia. Inform a senior immediately and make arrangements for emergency surgery.

POSTOPERATIVE PYREXIA

Normal body temperature is 36.7–37°C orally and 37.3–37.6°C rectally. Tympanic membrane temperature probes are equivalent to rectal temperature. There is a circadian rhythm for body temperature, with normal temperature being higher in the evening.

Postoperative pyrexia is usually, but not always, associated with infection. Do not start antibiotics blindly – always try to determine the possible causes of pyrexia and tailor therapy to the differential diagnosis. Do not forget to send specimens for microbiological examination prior to antibiotics. The most common causes are:

● Respiratory tract infections and atelectasis
● Superficial wound infection
● Deep infection/abscess
● Infection of indwelling lines
● Urinary tract infections
● DVT

Remember the **4 Ws**:

- **Wind** (respiratory tract)
- **Water** (UTI)
- **Wound**
- **Walking** (DVT)

See page 342 for pneumonia.

In general, pyrexia in the first 24 hours of elective surgery can be observed. If there has been pre-existing sepsis or faecal contamination during abdominal surgery, then the operating surgeon will usually prescribe postoperative antibiotic cover. Good postoperative analgesia and chest physiotherapy are useful for reducing the risk of atelectasis. **Note: A sharp rise in temperature within 36 hours after abdominal surgery associated with cardiovascular instability raises the possibility of leakage of bowel content or inadvertent bowel injury**. All patients with fever can become dehydrated quickly – adjust fluid input as guided by clinical signs of hydration, urine output, pulse and U&E.

Continuation of pyrexia, or pyrexia occurring after this period, requires thorough clinical evaluation to determine the likely source of infection. Table 1.7 summarises the usual temporal presentation of aetiologies. Blood and urine samples should be obtained for microbiological examination, and antibiotic therapy started empirically and changed in the light of clinical progress and antibiotic sensitivities. On auscultating the chest if there are signs of infection, obtain an X-ray and send any sputum specimens for culture. Note that green sputum makes pneumonia likely whereas clear sputum is equivocal.

Leakage from bowel anastomoses usually occurs after 3–5 days, although can occur at any time. This is associated with increasing abdominal pain, tachycardia, raised white cell count (WCC), metabolic acidosis, abdominal distension and prolonged ileus. This carries high mortality if intervention is delayed. Bear in mind the possibility of intra-abdominal sepsis in any patient who becomes unwell more than 3–5 days after a bowel surgery.

Pyrexia after a week should raise the possibility of a DVT. If the clinical signs for DVT are absent then consider investigating for a pulmonary embolus.

Table 1.7 Postoperative pyrexia

< 24 hours	Stress response to surgery Beware of bowel spillage Dissemination of pre-existing infection
24–72 hours	Pneumonia/atelectasis
> 3 days	Chest infection Wound infection Line infection Intraperitoneal sepsis/anastomotic leak Urinary tract infection
> 5 days	DVT/pulmonary embolism

Examination

- Temperature, pulse, blood pressure, urine output – hydration state
- Full physical examination – listen closely to the chest and look at the operation site
- Check Venflon sites for cellulitis
- Look at urine – cloudy?
- Look at sputum – green?
- Look at wounds
- Calf tenderness/leg swelling – evidence of DVT?

Investigations

- WCC, U&E
- Arterial blood gases (ABG) – check for acidosis
- Blood/urine/sputum/faecal culture
- Faeces for *Clostridium difficile* if there is diarrhoea
- Pus swab if any wound infection
- Ultrasound scan (USS)/computed tomography (CT) if deep infection/anastomotic leak suspected
- Deep vein duplex/ventilation-perfusion (V/Q) scan if DVT or pulmonary embolism (PE) suspected

All patients with chronic atrial fibrillation (INR 2.0–3.0) or patients with mechanical valves (INR 2.5–3.5) should be anticoagulated for life. Patients with a history of DVT, PE or atrial fibrillation that is expected to revert should be anticoagulated for a fixed period at the discretion of their team. The target INR is normally 2.0–3.0 for these conditions.

Postoperative (re-)warfarinisation usually starts on the first day unless contraindicated, and it is not necessary to prescribe a loading dose. If patients are already on warfarin prescribe the usual daily dose and adjust if necessary according to daily INR. For patients who are not on warfarin, prescribe 5 mg as a starting dose and adjust according to daily INR. The maintenance dose is usually 2–4 mg but special care should be exercised when initiating warfarin for patients with heart failure, liver disease or low body mass, when a lower starting dose is advisable. Check INR on day 2 but remember that warfarin has a delayed action and that the daily INR reflects the effect of warfarin given 2 days beforehand.

Table 1.8 Over-warfarinisation

Life-threatening haemorrhage	Give 1 mg vitamin K iv and 1000 ml fresh frozen plasma (FFP) stat
Non-life-threatening bleeding	Vitamin K 1 mg iv and review regularly
INR 4.5–7 without bleeding	Withhold warfarin and check INR daily
INR > 7 without bleeding	Withhold warfarin and consider vitamin K 1 mg iv

Note: Vitamin K comes in 10-mg ampoules but do not give more than 1 mg except in life-threatening haemorrhage because the patient will then be resistant to warfarin for weeks. In addition vitamin K will take at least 24 hours to work since the mechanism of action is through the synthesis of new clotting factors so in the presence of active bleeding intravenous clotting factor transfusion is the only treatment.

Patients who have new-onset postoperative atrial fibrillation and are not on warfarin should have LMWH coverage until cardioversion or warfarin treatment is established (INR > 2.0). After this time stop LMWH. Thromboembolic prophylaxis for heart valve surgery is summarised in Table 1.9.

Table 1.9 Anticoagulation and heart valve surgery

Procedure	Anticoagulation	Duration
All mechanical valves	Warfarin (INR 2.5–3.5)	Life
All tissue valves in sinus rhythm	Aspirin (75 mg)	Life
All valve repair in sinus rhythm	Aspirin (75 mg)	Life

HEPARIN THERAPY

Heparinisation may be necessary preoperatively in patients who are awaiting surgery but in whom the risk of thrombosis or thromboembolism necessitates continuing the infusion until surgery. Conversion to iv heparin is achieved by an initial bolus of 5000 IU unfractionated sodium heparin iv stat, followed by an infusion of 24 000–30 000 IU per 24 hours. It is essential to check the APTT every 6 hours and adjust the heparin dose to achieve an APTT ratio of 2–3. Incremental changes of 2000–3000 IU per 24 hours are used to adjust the APTT. Once a therapeutic APTT is achieved check the APTT ratio daily.

Fractionated heparin is unpredictable in its duration of action and is impossible to reverse so unfractionated heparin is often preferred.

Postoperative heparinisation is prescribed similarly until the INR is greater than 2. However, it is not uncommon for cardiac and vascular patients to be on a heparin infusion postoperatively, and this should be explained in the operative note. Often a 'therapeutic' dose of a LMWH given once a day by sc injection will suffice to fully anticoagulate such a patient. Again LMWH can be discontinued once the INR is ≥ 2.0.

GENERAL SURGERY

J GHOSH AND A J M WATSON

ABDOMINAL WALL INCISIONS

An abdominal incision (Figure 2.1) should:

- Allow good access into wound
- Be extendible if additional access is required
- Be safe and speedy to perform
- Be cosmetic

Figure 2.1 The most common abdominal incisions. See text for explanation

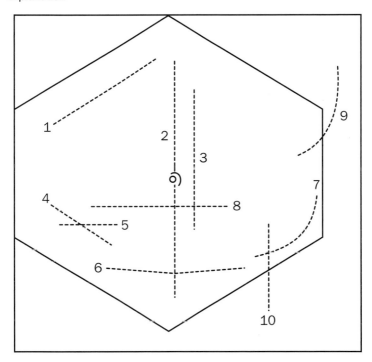

1. **Kocher's incision (right subcostal) for open cholecystectomy**

   - A reversed Kocher's incision may be made in left hypochondrium for elective splenectomy
   - A Kocher's and reverse Kocher's incision joined together in the midline creates a roof top or chevron incision and is commonly used for complex hepato-biliary or gastric surgery

2. **Midline incision through the linea alba**

   This is now the standard laparotomy approach and almost all intra-abdominal and retroperitoneal operations can be done using this approach. This may be upper (above the umbilicus), lower (below umbilicus) or long.

   Its advantages are:

   - Relatively little bleeding
   - No muscle division
   - No nerve division (which predisposes to hernia formation)
   - Quick
   - Extendible
   - Equal access to both sides of abdominal cavity

   Its main disadvantage is that it is more painful and thus can cause more ventilation compromise than a transverse approach, increasing risk of atelectasis, pneumonia and limiting mobility.

3. **Paramedian incision**

   Now rarely done. Located 2–3 cm lateral to the midline. Associated problems include:

   - Longer time required to create and close than midline incisions
   - May cause rectus abdominis atrophy leading to weakness
   - Limited access to contralateral structures

4. **Gridiron incision for appendicectomy**

   Allows good visualisation.

5. **Lanz incision**

   More cosmetic approach for appendicectomy than a gridiron incision.

6. Pfannenstiel incision

Standard gynaecological approach and used in prostate and bladder surgery. Usually located in the skin fold to improve cosmesis.

7. Rutherford–Morrison incision

Allows very good access into pelvis. Commonly used to place a transplanted kidney.

8. A transverse incision across the abdomen

This is being increasingly used for colonic and aortic surgery. It is advantageous as it causes less postoperative pain and a more cosmetic scar. It gives particularly good exposure in young children and short, obese adults. A transverse incision centred below the umbilicus is probably from a paraumbilical hernia repair. A small incision, around 2 cm long, just off the umbilicus indicates previous laparoscopic surgery.

9. Loin incision

For nephrectomy.

10. Vertical incision

Made to expose the common femoral artery, eg for femoro-popliteal bypass or femoro-femoral crossover. In the past this was also used for McEvedy's approach for femoral hernia repair, although now this is carried out through a transverse skin incision.

ABDOMINAL PAIN

Abdominal pain accounts for the majority of emergency general surgery workload and poses a challenge to surgeons at all levels. Assessment of a patient presenting with abdominal pain broadly has two objectives:

- To establish the degree of urgency and determine whether senior support is needed
- To list differential diagnoses (Table 2.1), create a management plan and to determine whether or not an operation is required

This is achieved by careful history taking, thorough examination and targeted investigations.

Table 2.1 Causes of abdominal pain (surgical emergencies highlighted in **bold**)

GENERALISED	CENTRAL
Aortic aneurysm	**Perforated ulcer**
Intestinal ischaemia	**Pancreatitis**
Visceral perforation	**Aortic aneurysm**
Intestinal obstruction	Cholecystitis
Sickle cell crisis	Gastritis
Diabetic ketoacidosis	Hepatitis
	Hepatic abscess

RIGHT UPPER QUADRANT	LEFT UPPER QUADRANT
Perforated ulcer	**Perforated ulcer**
Pancreatitis	**Aortic aneurysm**
Cholecystitis	**Pancreatitis**
Hepatitis	Gastritis
Gastritis	Pyelonephritis/renal stones
Hepatic abscess	**Boerhaave's syndrome**
Pyelonephritis/renal stones	
Right lower lobe lung disease	
High appendicitis	

RIGHT LOWER QUADRANT	LEFT LOWER QUADRANT
Aortic aneurysm	**Aortic aneurysm**
Pancreatitis	**Pancreatitis**
Caecal volvulus	**Sigmoid volvulus**
Ruptured ectopic pregnancy	**Ruptured ectopic pregnancy**
Appendicitis	Diverticulitis
Pyelonephritis/stones	Pyelonephritis/stones
Colon carcinoma	Colon carcinoma
Inflammatory bowel disease	Inflammatory bowel disease
Pelvic inflammatory disease	Pelvic inflammatory disease
Ovarian cyst	Ovarian cyst
Endometriosis	Endometriosis
Fibroid degeneration	Fibroid degeneration
Gynaecological tumour	Gynaecological tumour
Meckel's diverticulum	Meckel's diverticulum

History

It is important to take a detailed history of the pain itself – the SOCRATES acronym (Table 2.2) is useful for this.

Table 2.2 Questions regarding abdominal pain: **SOCRATES**

S	Site
O	Onset – sudden or gradual

C	Character
	   Severity
	   Constant/intermittent/colicky ('in waves' suggests obstruction of hollow viscus)

R	Radiation
	   Shoulder → subdiaphragmatic irritation, eg abscess or following laparoscopy
	   Right shoulder → cholecystitis
	   Back → pancreatitis, aortic aneurysm
	   Loin to groin → ureteric colic
	   Scrotum to groin → testicular torsion, orchitis

A	Associated symptoms
T	Time course (duration)

E	Exacerbating/relieving factors
	   Worse with movement → peritoneal irritation
	   Effect of food
	Association with menses

S	Systems review

Questions regarding pain

- Onset – sudden or gradual
- Duration
- Location
- Severity
- Nature – constant/intermittent/colicky/(pain occurring 'in waves' suggests obstruction of a hollow viscus)
- Radiation
- Shoulder → subdiaphragmatic irritation, eg abscess or following laparoscopy
- Right shoulder → cholecystitis
- Back → pancreatitis, aortic aneurysm

- Loin to groin → ureteric colic
- Scrotum to groin → testicular torsion, orchitis

Gastrointestinal symptoms

- Vomiting → obstruction
- Bowel habit/recent changes → colitis, carcinoma, gastroenteritis
- Weight loss → malignancy
- Jaundice

Urological/gynaecological symptoms

- Last menstrual period and regularity
- Per vaginal (PV) discharge → pelvic inflammatory disease (PID)
- Intrauterine contraceptive device
- Dysuria/urinary frequency/offensive urine → urinary tract infection

Other history

- Past medical history including cardiac, respiratory, diabetes, epilepsy, jaundice and sickle cell disease
- Detailed drug history needed but take special note of anticoagulation, non-steroidal anti-inflammatory drugs (NSAIDs), aspirin or steroid use
- Family history of inflammatory bowel disease or cancer
- Alcohol and smoking
- Independence at home and quality of life

Document last food and drink – in case general anaesthetic (GA) is needed.

Examination

- Always make a note of vital signs (pulse, blood pressure (BP), temperature, urine output) as they may be the first indication that senior support is needed. Pyrexia implies infective or inflammatory pathology. Tachycardia or hypotension suggests dehydration or shock. Urine output of ≤ 0.5 ml/kg per hour demonstrates hypovolaemia.
- General observation:

  ○ In pain?
  ○ Restless (colicky pain) or lying flat (peritonism)?
  ○ Clubbing
  ○ Jaundice (look at the sclerae – the 'whites of eyes')

○ Anaemia (look for general and conjunctival pallor)
○ Virchow's node (left supraclavicular lymph node – metastatic gastrointestinal malignancy)
○ Hydration (is the tongue dry?)
○ Abdomen

- Expose groins
- Scars
- Ask patient to cough → may show herniae, pain suggests peritonism
- Flat or swollen (remember the '**5 Fs**' as the causes of abdominal distension: **fat/fluid/faeces/flatus/fetus**)
- Site of tenderness
- Masses – deep or superficial? Pulsatile?
- Carefully check for organomegaly
- Hernial orifices – surprisingly easy to miss an irreducible femoral hernia
- Note Rovsing's and Psoas signs (see acute appendicitis section)

- **Guarding** is tensing of the abdominal wall on palpation. This is to 'guard' inflamed organs within the abdomen from the pain elicited by pressure.
- **Rebound tenderness** is pain felt when a hand pressing (gently) on the abdomen is suddenly released.
- **Peritonism** is localised abdominal pain on palpation associated with guarding and rebound tenderness. The remainder of the abdomen may be soft and non-tender. This indicates a local inflammatory process causing peritoneal irritation.
- **Peritonitis** is characterised by tenderness on light palpation associated with guarding and rebound tenderness affecting the whole of the abdomen. The abdominal wall is hard and the patient characteristically is fearful of any movement or pressure as this results in pain. The presence of peritonitis indicates an inflammatory process affecting the whole of the abdomen and invariably means urgent surgical intervention.
- Rectal examination – do not neglect this:

○ External – warts, anal cancer, skin tags, prolapse, piles, fissure
○ Internal – masses, note that an anterior mass in an elderly lady may be a pessary
○ Blood present – fresh or old?
○ Prostate

Investigations

- U&E, FBC, glucose, amylase, liver function tests (LFT) (particularly if jaundice or symptoms consistent with biliary cause)
- Pregnancy test – all women of child-bearing age
- Urine dipstick (and culture if positive)
- Erect CXR, abdominal X-ray (AXR)
- Group and save/crossmatch blood depending on whether there is bleeding and quantity of blood loss
- ABG and lactate – metabolic acidosis is suggestive of presence of serious pathology
- Further radiological investigations, eg USS or CT, may be required – discuss with senior

Treatment

Depends on underlying diagnosis. However, there are principles that should be followed in all patients presenting with acute abdominal pain.

The doctrine that opioid analgesia masks signs of peritonitis is antiquated, and there is no excuse for keeping a patient in pain while they are undergoing assessment. The patient should be kept nil by mouth until a differential diagnosis list and initial management plan is made. Intravenous access needs to be available and the patient hydrated with normal saline or Hartmann's solution. If the history indicates the need for a urinary catheter and/or nasogastric tube, then these should be prepared. For anybody with suspected peritonism, blood cultures need to be taken and broad-spectrum antibiotics (eg iv cefuroxime 750 mg tds and metronidazole 500 mg tds) started.

The following are **indicators of serious pathology** that require prompt senior review:

- Haemodynamic instability ($\uparrow$ pulse, $\downarrow$ blood pressure, $\downarrow$ urine output)
- Sepsis ($\uparrow$ temperature, $\uparrow$ WCC)
- Acidosis
- Pancreatitis ($\uparrow$ amylase)
- Pulsatile/expansile mass
- Guarding/peritonitis
- Gas under diaphragm on erect CXR (see pages 46–47)
- Intestinal distension on AXR (see page 47)

DIARRHOEA

The causes of diarrhoea are:

- Secretory
- Inflammatory – Crohn's disease, ulcerative colitis, radiation colitis, ischaemic colitis
- Infective – bacterial, viral, parasitic, amoebiasis
- *Campylobacter*, *Shigella*, *Escherichia coli* and *Salmonella* associated with bloody diarrhoea
- Malabsorption
- Increased bowel motility – irritable bowel syndrome, thyrotoxicosis, stimulant laxatives

C. DIFFICILE INFECTION

This is an increasingly common and life-threatening problem in surgical patients, especially elderly patients, and carries significant morbidity and mortality. Be highly suspicious of this in a patient with diarrhoea who is having, or has recently had, antibiotics.

C. difficile is a spore-forming, Gram-positive bacillus. Systemic antibiotics disrupt the normal colonic bacterial flora, facilitating *C. difficile* colonisation and growth. Both A and B enterotoxins from the bacillus elicit a release of pro-inflammatory cytokines, resulting in an inflammatory exudate on the colonic mucosal surface with intervening areas of normal mucosa – pseudomembranous colitis. The risk of *C. difficile* colonisation may persist for up to 2 months after antibiotic exposure.

History

Severe, persistent and watery diarrhoea associated with fever, dehydration and abdominal bloating.

Examination

Increasing abdominal pain, tenderness and sepsis suggests fulminant colitis or toxic dilatation. Oxygen/fluid resuscitation, AXR and senior review is needed – look for colonic dilatation.

Diagnosis is established from stool culture and enzyme-linked immunosorbent assay (ELISA) for enterotoxin A. The usual 'turnaround' time for this is 6–24 hours, although there will be a delay at weekends.

Treatment

- Stop current antibiotics – the diarrhoea often subsides with this. Liaise with microbiologists if this creates any difficulty with patient management. There will be hospital policies to cover infection control and barrier nursing
- Oral metronidazole 400 mg/8 hourly or vancomycin 125 mg/6 hourly
- Drugs causing constipation should be avoided
- There is a 20–30% relapse rate following metronidazole. Further course of antibiotic may be required after liaison with a microbiologist

---

METHODS OF REDUCING *C. DIFFICILE* RISK

- Optimising antibiotic use by close adherence to hospital antibiotic policies
- Ensuring personal and hospital cleanliness – this includes washing of hands between each patient encounter
- Isolation/cohort nursing of affected patients in available separate room – patients with diarrhoea may spread the infection to other patients

---

VOMITING

Causes of vomiting are:

- Gastrointestinal
  - Obstruction – when food is undigested and without bile, think gastric outflow obstruction or oesophageal stenosis
  - Gastroenteritis
  - Ileus/postoperative
  - Bowel obstruction

- Neurological causes

  ○ Raised intracranial pressure
  ○ Ménière's disease/labyrinthitis
  ○ Migraine

- Metabolic causes

  ○ Pregnancy
  ○ Renal failure and uraemia
  ○ Alcohol
  ○ Drugs, eg opioids

See section on intestinal obstruction/pseudo-obstruction.

X-RAY INTERPRETATION

ABDOMINAL X-RAY

- The standard AXR is taken with the patient lying in supine projection with X-rays projected from front to back (anteroposterior). When requesting an AXR, remember that radiation exposure of one plain AXR is equivalent to 50 CXRs – so ask yourself if it is necessary
- Next, as with all X-ray interpretations, make sure that you are looking at the correct patient's AXR and note the date that it was taken. For any plain X-ray, five densities may be found: (i) black represents (bowel) gas, (ii) white represents calcified structures such as bone, (iii) light grey represents soft tissue, (iv) darker grey represents fat, and (v) metallic objects such as staple lines or clips are seen as an intense bright white
- Check orientation and inspect x-ray systematically. Examine stomach in left upper quadrant. Examine small and large intestine gas pattern. If there is proximal dilatation think of gastric outflow obstruction whereas if there is global dilatation the obstruction is likely to be in the distal small bowel or colon. It is important to check for the presence of rectal gas as this may aid differentiation between obstruction and pseudo-obstruction
- Intraluminal gas should be described by its distribution and the diameter of intestine. Small and large intestines can be distinguished by luminal folds, particularly if the intestine is distended (Figure 2.2). The small intestine has mucosal folds

that cross the length of the lumen (plicae circularis/valvulae conniventes). This is particularly marked in the jejunum. The small bowel is classically centrally distributed. The large intestine has folds that do not cross the diameter of the lumen (haustrae) (Figure 2.3) and is typically seen at the periphery of the film. Faecal matter will only be seen in colon and rectum. Normally, the small intestine should be less that 3 cm in diameter, colon 6 cm and caecum no more than 12 cm

Figure 2.2 Small bowel distension. Note plicae circularis extending across the whole of the bowel diameter

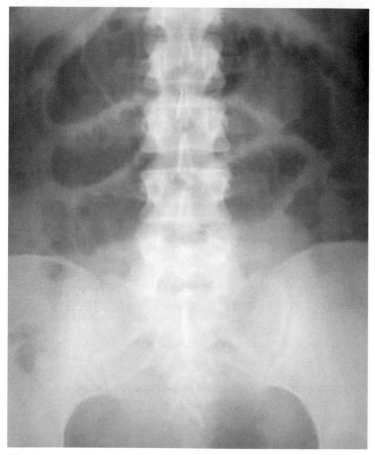

Figure 2.3 Large bowel obstruction demonstrating typical haustra pattern

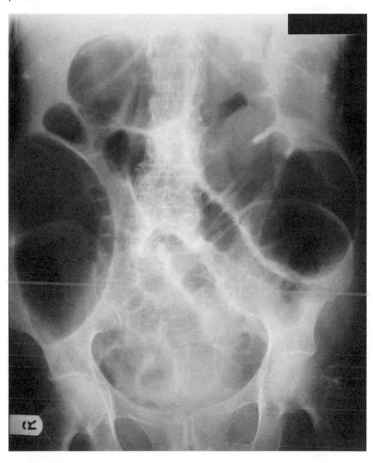

- To examine the urinary tract look at the L1 level for the renal pelvises (left higher than right) then track the ureters down the tips of the transverse processes, along the sacroiliac joint to the bladder shadow often visible above the pubis. Ninety per cent of renal/ureteric calculi are visible and only ten per cent of gallstones

- Calcified tissue can greatly aid diagnosis, such as calcified aorta or iliac vessels, suggesting ischaemic or aneurysmal pathology. There can also be calcification of the pancreas in chronic pancreatitis and calcification of uterine fibroids
- Air within the biliary tree may represent recent instrumentation (eg endoscopic retrograde cholangiopancreatography (ERCP)), a cholo-enteric fistula or ascending cholangitis
- Examination of bony tissue may reveal vertebral lytic (clear) or sclerotic (dense) lesions or arthritic changes

Figure 2.4 Erect CXR showing subdiaphragmatic air – highlighted by boxes

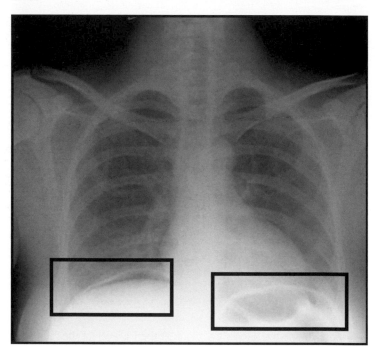

- eCXR allows visualisation of the lung fields and assessment of free gas in the peritoneal cavity (pneumoperitoneum). The latter is diagnosed by looking for air under the diaphragm (Figure 2.4)
- Free gas following perforation is seen under the diaphragm in an eCXR. An eCXR can detect as little as 1 ml of free air and has 95% specificity. However, it has lower sensitivity, with up to a third of perforations missed, if the X-ray is taken early
- Note that a subdiaphragmatic gastric gas bubble in the left upper quadrant is to be expected. A true pneumoperitoneum will follow the contour of the diaphragm closely, unlike a gastric gas bubble. Occasionally, a dilated loop of large bowel may confusingly appear like a pneumoperitoneum. If there is any doubt always check with a senior colleague or a radiologist. A lateral decubitus projection may be of help in difficult cases, with air visible over the liver
- The important point is that normal findings in an eCXR in a patient where there is clinical suspicion of a perforation do not exclude that possibility. Close monitoring of the patient and possibly repeated eCXR later in the day or during the following morning may be required

---

WHAT TO DO IF FREE GAS IS SEEN UNDER THE DIAPHRAGM

A pneumoperitoneum may be seen following perforation of a duodenal or gastric ulcer, small bowel perforation, or a large bowel perforation (due to malignancy, diverticulosis, strangulation or obstruction). It is a common (but not universal) observation that a small pneumoperitoneum arises from a gastric/duodenal perforation whereas a large volume of free gas suggests a colonic pathology.

Free abdominal gas usually means that a laparotomy is required to establish the diagnosis and to treat the underlying cause. Consequently, a senior needs to be involved early on. In the meantime the following actions may be instituted:

- Check whether there has been any recent abdominal surgery/laparoscopy
- Oxygen
- Ensure large-bore iv access and connect iv saline
- Urinary catheter with hourly measuring bag; maintain urine output of at least >0.5 ml/kg per hour
- Analgesia and anti-emetics
- Nasogastric tube with free drainage
- Nil by mouth; document when the patient last ate or drank
- Broad-spectrum antibiotics (eg cefuroxime 750 mg tds and metronidazole 500 mg tds)
- Make sure that blood results for U&E and FBC and group and save have been taken that day

ACUTE APPENDICITIS

Acute appendicitis affects 1 in 8 people. Right iliac fossa pain is a very common presenting symptom and establishing a diagnosis may be challenging particularly in women, due to the number of surgical, gynaecological and urological differential diagnoses. The diagnosis of acute appendicitis is made primarily on clinical grounds.

History

- Exact duration of pain – pain lasting continuously for longer than 3 days is less likely to be appendicitis
- Where did the pain start? Has it moved (central to right iliac fossa)?
- Onset of pain? Appendicitis is usually of gradual onset whereas a ruptured ovarian cyst has a sudden onset
- Any vomiting or nausea? Do you feel hungry (anorexia is associated with appendicitis)?
- Fever/sweats/rigours → infective pathology
- When was your last period? Are they regular? → risk of ectopic pregnancy

- Gynaecological history? PV discharge? → PID
- Burning urine? Blood in urine? → urinary tract infection (UTI)
- Does pain spread? Loin → ureteric stone; right shoulder → subdiaphragmatic pathology
- Recent 'flu-like illness/ENT infection? → mesenteric adenitis in young children
- Previous episodes

Examination

- Initially poorly localised, colicky central abdominal pain (visceral pain) for around 1 day
- Pain moves to right iliac fossa (Table 2.3) – centred at McBurney's point: junction of lateral third and medial two-thirds along a line between umbilicus and anterior superior iliac spine. Pain is now constant and associated with peritonism (peritoneal irritation as inflammation spreads to surrounding structures)
- Nausea, vomiting (developing regional ileus)
- Anorexia
- Lies still with pain (unlike ureteric colic)
- Pyrexia (usually mild 37.5–38°C. Can be higher with abscess formation)
- Tachycardia
- **Rovsing's sign** – pressure from left iliac fossa creates pain in right iliac fossa (pushes appendix against abdominal wall to illicit local tenderness)
- **Psoas sign**: right hip flexion against resistance (by placing a hand on patient's knee) results in pain due to iliopsoas irritation. Indicates retrocaecal, peri-psoas inflammation
- Rectal examination (do not neglect this in adult patients) – right pelvic pain associated with appendicitis. Cervical excitation associated with pelvic inflammatory disease and pelvic abscess

Investigations

- Raised WCC
- Pregnancy test in females to exclude ectopic pregnancy
- Abdominal X-ray has little role to play in diagnosing appendicitis. May be useful in excluding ureteric calculus
- Mid-stream urine (MSU) sample may be sent to exclude UTI. Urine dipstick may be positive in appendicitis
- C-reactive protein (CRP) will be raised but is non-specific

- Pelvic ultrasound scan is poorly sensitive but can identify gynaecological pathology
- CT scan is sensitive and specific, but not always readily available and delivers a relatively high radiation dose

Treatment

Keep patient nil by mouth, provide iv infusion and analgesia. Do not withhold analgesia in the fear of masking clinical signs. If a diagnosis of probable acute appendicitis has been reached and the decision to operate made, give iv broad-spectrum antibiotics (eg cefuroxime and metronidazole) while waiting for appendicectomy.

If diagnosis is equivocal, carry out active observation by taking note of temperature, observation and clinical signs every 4–6 hours. Acute appendicitis usually becomes more obvious with time. If symptoms persist and the diagnosis is still not clear after 24 hours, a pelvic USS or diagnostic laparoscopy is useful. Despite these measures, up to 20% of appendicectomies will turn out to be normal. Diagnostic laparoscopy, despite the need for a GA, has the advantage of direct visualisation of the appendix and pelvic organs and concomitant laparoscopic appendicectomy.

Following appendicectomy, most patients will be able to start oral intake during the first postoperative day and are ready to be discharged when mobile and comfortable. This is prolonged if there has been perforation and pelvic contamination with pus. If the appendix has been found to be perforated then continue broad-spectrum antibiotics (eg cefuroxime and metronidazole) until sepsis resolves. Remember to use DVT prophylaxis.

Table 2.3 Causes of right iliac fossa pain

GI/vasular	Gynaecological	Urological
Appendicitis	Ruptured ectopic pregnancy	Referred testicular pain
Ileitis	Ruptured ovarian cyst	UTI
Cholecystitis	Pelvic inflammatory disease	Ureteric stone
Groin hernia	Acute salpingitis	
Iliac artery aneurysm	Endometriosis	

APPENDIX MASS

An appendix mass forms following perforation of an inflamed appendix, which becomes walled off by an adherent covering of omentum and small bowel. This typically occurs 2–5 days after onset of symptoms. The history is similar to that of appendicitis with a longer duration.

Examination reveals a mass in the right iliac fossa and pyrexia. The clinical diagnosis is confirmed by either USS or CT. A caecal tumour must be excluded, particularly in elderly patients.

Conventionally, treatment involves conservative treatment with broad-spectrum antibiotics until there is clinical evidence of improvement. This is usually followed by an elective interval appendicectomy after 6 weeks to 3 months. Non-resolving cases may require percutaneous drainage of pus.

MECKEL'S DIVERTICULUM

A Meckel's diverticulum represents the remains of the vitello-intestinal duct. It is a true diverticulum (ie all layers of bowel wall) of the anti-mesenteric border of ileum and is remembered by the **rule of 2s**:

- Present in 2% of the population
- 2 feet from ileocaecal junction
- 2 inches long
- 2 male: 1 female ratio

Meckel's diverticulitis may mimic appendicitis. If a normal appendix is found during appendicectomy, a Meckel's diverticulum must be looked for. Although most are asymptomatic, ulceration of ectopic gastric mucosa may cause bleeding (sometime presenting as rectal bleeding), abdominal pain or perforation with peritonitis.

With the recognition of *Helicobacter pylori* and the introduction of H_2 receptor antagonists and proton pump inhibitors (PPIs), the incidence of perforated peptic ulcers has fallen dramatically. However, due to the widespread use of NSAIDs and steroids, as well as the high prevalence of alcohol misuse, this remains a relatively common presentation. Although 80% of patients with a perforated peptic ulcer have a preceding history of dyspepsia, perforation while on PPI is uncommon.

During the first 6 hours, there is an acute onset of upper/general abdominal pain which is worse with movement and may radiate to the shoulders (subdiaphragmatic irritation). This is not initially associated with signs of sepsis, as the early chemical peritonitis is usually relatively pathogen free. As peritoneal contamination progresses, the pain escalates and becomes associated with sepsis (raised WCC and temperature). The patient has no appetite but vomiting is usually not a feature. There may be associated melaena.

History
- Onset of pain – slow onset unlikely to be perforated ulcer
- Constant or colicky?
- Worse with movement?
- Radiation to shoulder?
- History of abdominal pain or heartburn?
- Alcohol or cigarette use?
- Drug history – NSAIDs, aspirin or steroids? PPI?

Examination
- Upper/generalised abdominal tenderness
- Guarding and rebound tenderness
- Reduced bowel sounds
- Make sure there is no abdominal aortic aneurysm (AAA)
- Patient does not want to be moved

Investigations
- U&E, FBC, group and save
- Amylase – may be mildly raised
- eCXR (see AXR and eCXR sections above, pages 43–46)

Treatment

- Prepare for laparotomy and omental patch repair
- Oxygen and fluid resuscitation
- iv PPI
- Nasogastric tube on free drainage
- iv broad-spectrum antibiotics
- Analgesia

GASTROINTESTINAL OBSTRUCTION

Bowel obstruction may be characterised as functional (paralytic ileus) or mechanical. In varying degrees, all types of bowel obstruction will be associated with four classic features:

- Colicky abdominal pain – coincides with peristaltic waves
- Abdominal swelling – more pronounced with distal obstruction
- Vomiting – profuse with proximal obstruction, later onset with distal obstruction
- Absolute constipation (of faeces and flatus)

When assessing any patient with bowel obstruction, the aim is to determine:

- Is this functional (paralytic ileus) or mechanical?
- Small or large bowel obstruction?
- Is there ischaemic bowel?
- Is there one or several points of obstruction?
- Underlying causes?

Each of these affects the management plan.

> The following points under History, Examination, Investigations and Treatment apply to all cases of clinical bowel obstruction. Specific points regarding small and large bowel obstruction as well as pseudo-obstruction are addressed in turn below.

History

- Previous abdominal/pelvic surgery? Previous malignancy? Scars present?
- Previous abdominal sepsis or irradiation?

- Preceding changes in bowel habit or constitutional symptoms (eg weight loss)
- Vomiting undigested food → gastric outflow obstruction

Examination

- Hyperactive 'tinkling' (mechanical obstruction) or absent bowel sounds (ileus or long-standing mechanical obstruction)?
- Groin swellings? → incarcerated hernia
- Do not forget to do a digital rectal examination to assess for rectal or pelvic masses, or a capacious rectum associated with pseudo-obstruction

Investigations

- U&E – electrolyte disturbance, particularly hypokalaemia
- FBC – ↑ WCC, ↓ Hb
- ABG and lactate – metabolic acidosis
- AXR
- Amylase – exclude pancreatitis, although also elevated to smaller degree with bowel ischaemia

Treatment

- Oxygen
- Large-bore iv access
- Intravenous rehydration – assessment made by pulse/BP/urine output monitoring, and serial U&E
- Urinary catheter with close fluid balance and electrolyte control
- Nil by mouth and nasogastric tube with free drainage to decompress small bowel and avoid aspiration
- Intravenous analgesia
- Intravenous broad-spectrum antibiotics (eg cefuroxime 750 mg tds and metronidazole 500 mg tds) following blood culture if clinically septic
- DVT prophylaxis

PARALYTIC ILEUS

Occurs with impaired bowel motility and is often associated with recent abdominal surgery, sepsis, fluid and electrolyte derangement (particularly hypokalaemia) and use of opioid analgesia (Table 2.4). The small bowel is predominantly affected.

Table 2.4 Causes of paralytic ileus

Local	Systemic
Post-operative	Pneumonia
Peritonitis	Uraemia
Retroperitoneal haematoma	Spinal injury
Abscess	Ketoacidosis
Pancreatitis	Hypercalcaemia
Abdominal trauma	Burns
Mesenteric ischaemia/infarction	Hypokalaemia
	Sepsis
	Jaundice
	Opioids

History

Abdominal distension, absolute constipation and nausea/vomiting are typically more prominent features than pain.

Examination

Dilated abdomen, absent bowel sounds, faeculent (not 'faecal'!) vomitus. Severe pain or guarding suggests either that an alternative pathology is present or that the bowel has become ischaemic.

Investigations

Ileus progression is determined predominantly on clinical grounds and with serial AXRs. A water-soluble contrast study is useful if there is doubt whether the obstruction is functional or mechanical – free flow of contrast is seen with paralytic ileus or incomplete mechanical obstruction. If there is a history of recent gastrointestinal surgery and evidence of sepsis, consider the possibility of an intra-abdominal collection – investigated by USS or CT. Remember to check for *C. difficile*.

Treatment

Initial resuscitation as above. Identification of an underlying aetiology allows resolution by 2–4 days in most cases. Prolonged ileus raises concern of either an unrecognised mechanical obstruction or continued physiological insult or source of sepsis.

SMALL BOWEL OBSTRUCTION

Mechanical bowel obstruction is most commonly due to adhesions following previous abdominal or pelvic surgery (60% cases). However other causes such as malignancies (20%) and herniae (10%) must be considered. The causes of small bowel obstruction (Table 2.5) include luminal occlusion (usually at the ileo-caecal valve), mural disease or extraluminal compression.

Table 2.5 Causes of small bowel obstruction

Lumen	Mural	Extramural
Food bolus	Caecal carcinoma	Adhesions
Gallstone ileus	Small bowel tumour	Herniae
Bezoars	Lymphoma	Volvulus
	Crohn's disease	Congenital band
	Intussusception	
	Radiation injury	
	Fibrous stricture	

History

Colicky abdominal pain maximal centrally and vomiting are predominant. Abdominal distension and absolute constipation may be limited in very proximal obstruction.

Investigations

Water-soluble contrast follow-through to distinguish between ileus, incomplete and complete obstruction. CT scan also gives similar information and may identify a causative aetiology.

Treatment

- Initial resuscitation as above
- Nasogastric tube, 'drip and suck' and replace high nasogastric losses with normal saline with potassium
- Treat any identifiable cause (eg hernia incarceration)
- Laparotomy is necessary if there is evidence of bowel ischaemia or non-resolution with conservative treatment
- Senior review is mandatory and ideally the patient should be observed within a HDU environment

LARGE BOWEL OBSTRUCTION

Carcinoma (50%), volvulus (15%) and diverticular disease (10%) are predominant causes. Less common causes are extrinsic compression from a malignancy, faecal impaction and benign stricture. Caecal perforation can ensue if large bowel obstruction is not relieved, due to its disproportionately large diameter (based on Laplace's Law). Therefore, always note the caecal diameter on the AXR.

Incompetence of the ileo-caecal valve (20% of cases), ie retrograde transit of colonic gas into the small bowel, reduces the risk of perforation by allowing decompression of the caecum. Valve incompetence is revealed in AXR by co-existence of large and small bowel distension.

History
Colicky abdominal pain, maximal centrally and in the lower abdomen, abdominal distension and absolute constipation are predominant. Vomiting classically occurs later.

Examination
Warning signs of an impending caecal perforation:

- Caecal maximal diameter greater than 14 cm on AXR
- Right iliac fossa tenderness

Impending caecal perforation is an indication for laparotomy. Senior help should be sought immediately and the patient ideally observed in the HDU setting.

Investigations
A single-contrast Gastrografin enema or CT scan will differentiate between ileus and mechanical obstruction.

Treatment
- Initial resuscitation as above
- Laparotomy if there is threatened bowel perforation or treatable underlying cause

VOLVULUS

A volvulus is an abnormal rotation of colon (sigmoid 75%, caecum 25% of cases) on its suspending mesentery resulting in complete or incomplete luminal occlusion and venous ischaemia. It is commonly seen in elderly patients, often those who are institutionalised with confusional states, dementia or psychiatric disorders. Patients often have a previous history of similar problems – 50% of sigmoid volvulus will recur.

History and examination

- Acute large bowel obstruction (see page 57) – abdominal distension is often gross
- Previous history
- May present with symptoms and signs suggestive of bowel ischaemia (see pages 67–69)

Investigations

- U&E, FBC, crossmatch blood
- ABG
- The diagnosis of a sigmoid volvulus is made on AXR, although caecal volvulus is usually found at laparotomy
- A single-contrast enema is very useful in confirming the diagnosis. A 'bird's beak' is seen at the distal end of the volvulus

---

INDICATIONS THAT THE BOWEL IS ISCHAEMIC AND NEEDS SURGERY

- Increasing abdominal pain with tenderness and peritonism
- Tachycardia
- ↑ WCC
- Metabolic acidosis

Treatment

Initial treatment of a sigmoid volvulus is resuscitation as described above and flatus tube decompression provided that there is little evidence of imminent perforation (see box above). The flatus tube is passed per rectum via a rigid sigmoidoscope to decompress the point of torsion which allows the volvulus to unwind. It is usually left for a minimum of 48 hours. Laparotomy is necessary following failed flatus tube decompression, recurrence, signs of imminent perforation or caecal volvulus.

Surgical treatment of a sigmoid volvulus is classically a Paul Mikulicz 'double-barrel' stoma, where the volvulus is resected and the two ends of bowel brought to the skin as stomas placed side by side. This allows easy stoma reversal at a later date. Hartmann's operation (sigmoid colectomy with an end proximal colostomy and rectal stump left in the pelvis) is also done where bowel is unhealthy and the distal stump cannot be brought superficially. Resection and anastomosis is not commonly done as an emergency procedure due to ischaemia increasing the risk of anastomosis failure.

Caecal volvulus is treated by a right hemicolectomy with either stoma formation or primary anastomosis (since blood supply here is superior to the left side of the colon).

DIVERTICULITIS

Diverticulosis is the presence of diverticula (outpouchings of the colonic mucosa through colon wall), most commonly found in the sigmoid colon. It is rare in patients younger than 40 years, but present in 40% of those over 60 years and increases in prevalence with age. **Acute diverticulitis** is acute infection within a diverticulum. Non-resolving diverticulitis may result in abscess, phlegmon (inflammatory mass), stricture or perforation. The differential diagnosis of acute diverticulitis includes:

- Colorectal carcinoma
- Crohn's disease
- Ulcerative colitis
- Ischaemic colitis

History

Acute diverticulitis starts with gradual lower abdominal pain (visceral pain) moving to the left iliac fossa (somatic pain) associated with accompanying fever and sweats. It has thus been described as a 'left-sided appendicitis'. It may be associated with diarrhoea or constipation.

Examination

- Pyrexia
- Localised peritonism in the left iliac fossa
- Perforated diverticulum associated with peritonitis
- Phlegmon and abscess may be associated with a left iliac fossa mass and local peritonism

Investigations

- WCC, Hb, CRP
- U&E
- Amylase – to exclude pancreatitis as differential diagnosis
- ABG – acidosis
- eCXR – exclude perforation
- AXR – exclude obstruction
- CT abdomen – the gold standard to establish diagnosis and determine the presence of any complications of diverticulitis
- Barium enema and colonoscopy inadvisable in acute setting due to risk of perforation

Treatment

Uncomplicated diverticula merely require a high-fibre diet.

All diverticulitis

- Nil by mouth and iv infusion
- Intravenous broad-spectrum antibiotics (eg cefuroxime and metronidazole)
- DVT prophylaxis
- Urinary catheter and monitor urinary output

Localised abscess without peritonitis

- CT-guided percutaneous drainage

Perforation and peritonitis

- Laparotomy is required; thus an early anaesthetic input
- Need fluid resuscitation
- Broad-spectrum antibiotics
- Group and save
- Inform HDU/ITU for postoperative recovery

COMPLICATIONS OF DIVERTICULOSIS

- Bleeding
- Acute diverticulitis
- Perforation and peritonitis
- Abscess
- Phlegmon (inflammatory mass)
- Stricture and large bowel obstruction
- Fistula (eg colo-vesical fistula)

INFLAMMATORY BOWEL DISEASE

Inflammation of the gastrointestinal tract may occur in:

- Crohn's disease
- Ulcerative colitis
- Infection
- Radiation enteritis
- Ischaemic colitis
- Drug-induced colitis

This section focuses on Crohn's disease and ulcerative colitis.

CROHN'S DISEASE

- A chronic inflammatory disorder which may affect any part of the gastrointestinal tract
- 30%: small bowel involvement only – especially terminal ileum
- 40%: large and small bowel involvement
- 50%: perianal involvement – fistulae, abscesses, skin tags, fissures

Crohn's disease patients have recurrent attacks, with acute 'flares' of the disease interspersed with periods of remission or less active disease. The inflammation affects all layers of the intestinal wall and is focal (unlike ulcerative colitis). Inflammatory regions may be separated by normal segments of bowel ('skip lesions'). Incidence 5–6/100 000, females > males; peak incidence 25–40 years (small peak in 60s); family history may be present.

Urgent presentations

Local perforation

- Pain and peritonism
- Sepsis (fever, tachycardia, ↑ WCC, acidosis)

Generalised peritonitis

- Pain and peritonitis
- Sepsis
- May have free gas on eCXR

Toxic dilatation

- Pain and peritonism
- Sepsis
- Dilated bowel on AXR

Complications

- Obstruction (chronic fibrosis)
- Abscess
- Perforation
- Fistula (eg entero-enteric, entero-cutaneous, entero-vesical)
- Toxic dilatation leading to perforation
- Bleeding
- Malignant change in chronic cases
- Gallstones (disrupted biliary metabolism with terminal ileal disease)
- Extra-intestinal manifestations in 15% (see Table 2.6)

History

Acute presentation:

- Abdominal pain → seen in acute inflammation, stricture, perforation, toxic dilatation. Pain can also be due to adhesions from previous surgery → common in patients with long-standing Crohn's

- Diarrhoea → colitis. Establish frequency of stools
- Bloody diarrhoea → colitis
- Mucus per rectum → colitis
- Systemic symptoms – fever, malaise, weight loss
- Vomiting → obstruction
- Perianal pain/discharge → perianal involvement

Other important questions:

- Duration of disease
- Previous surgery and anatomical location of previous episodes
- Maintenance therapy and normal baseline symptoms
- Symptoms of extra-intestinal manifestations (Table 2.6)
- Family history

Examination

- Temperature, pulse and BP → dehydration, sepsis
- Abdominal tenderness → guarding or peritonitis suggests perforation or toxic dilatation
- Mass → more common in right iliac fossa (terminal ileum). Suggests inflammatory mass and/or local perforation
- Distension – suggests obstruction or toxic dilatation
- Bowel sounds: if hyperactive → obstruction, if absent → perforation, abscess or toxic dilatation
- Note evidence of previous surgery – scars, stoma
- Perianal examination – look for abscess, skin tags, fissure, external fistula opening (may be discharging pus). Unless excessively tender, carry out a rectal examination to look for blood, masses and evidence of perianal disease

Investigations

- U&E – dehydration, ↓ K$^+$
- FBC – ↓ Hb, ↑ WCC
- CRP and erythrocyte sedimentation rate (ESR) – markers of inflammation
- Amylase – exclusion of pancreatitis as a differential diagnosis
- ABG – acidosis suggests intra-abdominal sepsis or fulminant inflammation
- AXR/eCXR – obstruction, toxic dilatation, perforation
- Stool culture – exclude infective cause
- CT scan – request if perforation is suspected but not seen in X-ray, mass is felt or if abscess is suspected

- Barium small bowel follow through – to visualise small bowel. Will show mucosal inflammation, stricture (string sign of Kantor) and fistula
- Barium enema – to visualise colon. Will show presence of mucosal inflammation, stricture or fistulae
- Flexible sigmoidoscopy/colonoscopy – allow direct visualisation and biopsy if diagnosis in doubt. Avoid if there is suspected obstruction, toxic dilation or perforation

Treatment

Oxygen and fluid resuscitation. Plus:

Medical

- Systemic steroids, eg prednisolone, hydrocortisone
- Topical steroids (Predfoam enema) – proctitis
- Mesalazine – for colitis
- Immunomodulators (azathioprine/ciclosporin) – resistant cases
- Infliximab (monoclonal antibody that neutralises tumour necrosis factor alpha (TNF-α)) for non-healing perianal fistula, severe Crohn's disease resistant to other treatment
- Nutrition – enteric feed or total parenteral nutrition (TPN) as appropriate; liaise with dietician

In event of fistula, this is treated by maintaining hydration, nutrition (may need TPN), reducing sepsis (broad-spectrum antibiotics and drainage of any abscess) and reducing secretions (eg oral fluid restriction, codeine, loperamide, octreotide and PPIs).

Surgical

Surgery is required if there is perforation, abscess, stricture, non-healing fistula or malignant change.

In the event of a perforation:

- Nil by mouth
- Fluid resuscitation, give oxygen
- IV antibiotics
- Urinary catheter and maintain urine output > 0.5 ml/kg per hour
- Laparotomy needed ASAP – inform senior

In event of toxic dilatation:

- Nil by mouth
- Fluid resuscitation, give oxygen
- Urinary catheter and maintain urine output >0.5 ml/kg per hour
- Full medical treatment including iv systemic steroids, iv broad-spectrum antibiotics, DVT prophylaxis
- Consult gastroenterologists
- Active observations including hourly observation and regular abdominal examination; serial daily AXR

Warning signs that laparotomy is needed

- Guarding/peritonism, increasing distension, sepsis

Table 2.6 Extra-intestinal features of inflammatory bowel disease

Related to disease activity	Unrelated to disease activity
Pyoderma gangrenosum	Sacroiliitis/ankylosing spondylitis
Erythema nodosum	Fatty liver
Aphthous ulcer	Chronic active hepatitis/cirrhosis
Arthropathy/arthritis	Primary sclerosing cholangitis
	Cholangiocarcinoma/hepatoma
	Gall stones/kidney stones
	Amyloidosis
	Clubbing
	Conjunctivitis/Uveitis/Episcleritis

ULCERATIVE COLITIS

Recurrent inflammatory disorder always affecting the rectum and often the colon. Inflammation is continuous, so 'skip lesions' are not found (unlike Crohn's).

Incidence 10–15/10 000, male = female, peak incidence 20–40 years. Up to 30% have extra-intestinal manifestations (see Table 2.6).

History

- Blood/mucus per rectum + diarrhoea – establish frequency of stools
- Anal irritation
- Systemic symptoms – fever, malaise, weight loss

Other important questions:

- Duration of disease
- Maintenance therapy and normal baseline bowel habit
- Symptoms of extra-intestinal manifestations (see Table 2.6)

Examination

- U&E – dehydration, $\downarrow K^+$
- FBC – $\downarrow$ Hb, $\uparrow$ WCC
- CRP and ESR – markers of inflammation
- LFT – $\downarrow$ albumin
- Amylase – exclusion of pancreatitis as a differential diagnosis
- ABG – acidosis suggests intra-abdominal sepsis or fulminant inflammation
- AXR/erect CXR – obstruction, toxic dilatation, perforation. Toxic megacolon should be suspected if colon diameter > 6 cm
- CT scan – request if abscess is suspected
- Barium enema – 'lead-pipe' colon → contracted pelvis; loss of haustra patterns → pseudopolyps
- Colonoscopy can confirm diagnosis, extent and allow biopsy. Avoid if toxic dilation is suspected

Treatment

Medical

- Steroids – topical (Predfoam) for local control of proctitis, or systemic (hydrocortisone, prednisolone) if there is severe colitis or concern of toxic dilatation
- 5-Acetylsalicylic acid (ASA) – mesalazine or sulfasalazine
- Broad-spectrum antibiotics if toxic dilatation or fulminant colitis

Surgical

- Laparotomy and subtotal colectomy/panproctocolectomy – indicated if there is toxic megacolon, perforation, failure to respond to medical treatment or severe bleeding
- Assessment and treatment of toxic colonic dilatation is as described for Crohn's disease. Be sure that the patent is well hydrated, oxygenated, on steroids and broad-spectrum antibiotics. The patient must be examined regularly (every 1–4 hours) and any progressing peritonism or systemic sepsis should be considered as warning for impending perforation and requirement for laparotomy

GASTROINTESTINAL ISCHAEMIA

Intestinal ischaemia may occur from arterial (more common) or venous occlusion (Table 2.7). Acute arterial occlusion results in rapid necrosis of the bowel wall, with the mucosa being most sensitive to hypoxia. Conversely, chronic ischaemia runs a more indolent course due to the gradual development of collateral vessels. Symptoms from chronic ischaemia develop whenever oxygen demand exceeds that supplied by the collateral circulation, often seen during digestion of food.

Table 2.7 Causes of intestinal ischaemia

Acute arterial ischaemia	Chronic arterial ischaemia	Venous ischaemia
Atherosclerosis Embolism Extrinsic compression (eg strangulated hernia) Arterial spasm Prolonged hypotension (eg following trauma) Iatrogenic (eg aortic cross clamping)	Atherosclerosis Vasculitis (eg polyarteritis nodosa)	Thrombosis secondary to hypercoagulability (eg polycythemia) Bowel wall dilatation

History

Acute intestinal ischaemia classically presents with severe pain with relatively few signs on clinical examination.

Chronic intestinal ischaemia presents with an indolent course of post-prandial abdominal pain ('intestinal angina'), associated anorexia ('food fear'), weight loss and diarrhoea.

Examination

The abdomen is classically 'soft and silent'. Relatively few signs are elicited, given the severity of pain. Acute ischaemia caused by emboli may be associated with the diagnostic triad:

- Severe abdominal pain
- Diarrhoea and vomiting
- Cardiac disease as a source of emboli

Investigations

Diagnosis is often made on clinical suspicion as laboratory tests are poorly specific.

- Raised WCC, metabolic acidosis, raised serum lactate and moderately raised amylase are all associated findings
- eCXR to exclude perforation
- AXR may show bowel distension and intestinal wall thickening (thumb-printing)
- Mesenteric angiography is diagnostic for arterial ischaemia, but is often not readily available
- CT with iv contrast and MRI are the gold standards for mesenteric venous thrombosis

Treatment

A high index of suspicion is required for timely diagnosis. Resuscitation requires:

- Oxygen via mask
- Intravenous rehydration
- Urinary catheter
- Nasogastric tube

If a strong suspicion of acute intestinal ischaemia is present, a diagnostic laparoscopy/laparotomy is the only way to establish the diagnosis. The prognosis is bleak with up to 90% mortality if diagnosis is delayed. Senior review is required rapidly to determine need for operative intervention.

GASTROINTESTINAL BLEEDING

In the acute setting, concurrent with clinical assessment institute simultaneous oxygen and fluid resuscitation. Judge whether there is clinical evidence of hypovolaemia. Evidence of hypovolaemia or active bleeding requires urgent senior review.

SIGNS OF HYPOVOLAEMIA

- Tachycardia
- Hyperventilation
- Hypotension
- Clamminess
- Reduced conscious level
- Reduced urine output
- Reduced capillary refill time

UPPER GASTROINTESTINAL BLEEDING

CAUSES OF UPPER GASTROINTESTINAL BLEEDING

- Duodenal ulcer (from underlying gastroduodenal artery) – majority
- Oesophageal varices (look for signs of liver disease)
- Gastric ulcer/gastritis
- Oesophagitis
- Malignancy
- Mallory–Weiss tear (following forceful vomiting)
- Portal hypertensive gastropathy
- Aorto-duodenal fistula
- Dieulafoy's ulcer (vascular malformation 2–5 cm distal to gastro-oesophageal junction)

History

- Melaena (80% cases) – note that as little as 50 ml of blood may cause melaena
- Haematemesis (bright or 'coffee-ground' vomit)
- Haematochezia (bright blood per rectum) – only if bleeding very brisk
- Classically bleeding distal to the splenic flexure of the colon generates bright rectal bleeding
- Collapse
- Symptoms of anaemia

Useful questions to ask:

- Estimated volume of blood loss
- Previous gastric/aortic surgery
- Previous symptoms of heartburn or epigastric pain
- NSAID/aspirin/steroid use $\rightarrow$ duodenal/gastric ulcer
- Alcohol misuse/liver disease $\rightarrow$ varices
- Anticoagulation/antiplatelet drugs/clopidogrel
- Recent vomiting $\rightarrow$ Mallory–Weiss tear
- Weight loss or jaundice $\rightarrow$ malignancy
- Age $\rightarrow$ malignancy more common in elderly patients

Examination

- Evidence of hypovolaemia, as above
- Hepatomegaly/stigmata of hepatic disease $\rightarrow$ varices
- Epigastric mass $\rightarrow$ malignancy
- Virchow's node (left supraclavicular lymph node) $\rightarrow$ gastrointestinal malignancy
- Previous abdominal surgery
- Epigastric pain $\rightarrow$ ulcer

Investigations

- FBC and clotting
- LFT – liver disease/metastasis
- Urea/creatinine (mmol/l) ratio >100 suggests upper gastrointestinal bleed as digested blood raises urea
- Group and save/crossmatch blood
- Gastroscopy >95% sensitive in finding cause – all patients should have oesophago-gastroduodenoscopy (OGD) within 24 hours. The urgency of this depends upon the extent of bleeding. Gastroscopy can also be used therapeutically

- Angiography is beneficial to elucidate the site of active bleeding but blood loss of > 0.5 ml/min is required to visualise a bleeding point and is not readily available in many units
- Nasogastric aspirate and barium swallow have a high false-negative rate

Treatment

Institute resuscitation as required:

- Oxygen
- Two large bore peripheral Venflon – at least 18 gauge (green)
- Intravenous rehydration. If patient is haemodynamically stable with normal BP and pulse, then crystalloid fluids are sufficient. If there is evidence of hypovolaemia, then colloids or blood is required, with senior colleague input
- Urinary catheter to monitor hourly urine output (maintain at > 5 ml/kg per hour)
- Start iv PPIs

Gastroscopy required to determine source of bleeding (oesophageal varices, gastric or duodenal bleeding) and to intervene. The timing of intervention depends on the degree of instability of patient; continued bleeding and hypovolaemia not improving with fluid resuscitation need senior review and urgent gastroscopy.

Variceal bleeding can be treated initially with a Sengstaken tube. This is a double-lumen tube that allows tamponade of the distal oesophagus and suction of gastric contents. Vasopressin and octreotide are also of benefit, as directed by a senior.

Gastric/duodenal bleeding may be controlled by 1:10 000 adrenaline injected into the base and edges of the bleeding ulcer. Other endoscopic treatments include cryotherapy, alcohol injection, saline injection, clipping and argon beam coagulation.

Failure of above management necessitates surgery, eg oversewing of ulcer or gastrectomy.

LOWER GASTROINTESTINAL BLEEDING

CAUSES OF BLEEDING PER RECTUM

Colorectal

- Diverticulosis
- Colorectal carcinoma
- Adenomatous polyp
- Proctocolitis (Crohn's disease, ulcerative colitis, irradiation, infective)
- Angiodysplasia
- Ischaemic bowel

Anal

- Haemorrhoids
- Fissure-in-ano
- Carcinoma of anus

Other

- Massive upper gastrointestinal bleed
- Meckel's diverticulum
- Aorto-enteric fistula

History

- Haematemesis is always absent if bleeding arises from lower GI tract
- Haematochezia
- Melaena if proximal bleeding source
- Collapse
- Symptoms of anaemia
- Note that 80% of lower gastrointestinal bleeds stop spontaneously and so unless the bleeding is heavy, persistent or causing haemodynamic disturbance, invasive investigations can be delayed

Useful questions:

- Bright or dark blood?
- Mucus/slime present? → inflammatory bowel disease
- How is the blood noticed – blood mixed in or separate to stools? Blood streak on paper?
- Mucus with stools?
- Past or family history of gastrointestinal disease?
- Anal or abdominal pain?
- Disturbance of bowel habit? Clarify the frequency and consistency of stools
- Recent weight loss? Lethargy?
- Fever/night sweats?

Table 2.8 Some classic patterns of lower gastrointestinal bleeding

Massive bleeding	Classically due to diverticular disease or angiodysplasia
Bright blood streaking tissue paper	Associated with anal pathology
Painful bright rectal bleeding	Associated with fissure-in-ano
Blood mixed in stool	Usually from proximal colon
Blood with mucus, diarrhoea and fever	Associated with inflammatory bowel disease or gastroenteritis
Preceding weight loss, altered bowel habit, abdominal pain	Associated with colorectal cancer or inflammatory bowel disease

Investigations

- FBC, crossmatch blood if severe bleeding
- Check clotting
- U&E – hypokalaemia with mucus-secreting polyps or if there is a history of diarrhoea
- LFT (to look for liver metastases) and carcinoembryonic antigen (CEA) (colorectal tumour marker) if suspicion of cancer exists
- Urea/creatinine (mmol/l) ratio < 100
- Invasive investigations aim to localise the site of bleeding and determine aetiology:

- ○ Flexible sigmoidoscopy/colonoscopy – allows direct visualisation of site and cause of bleeding. Endoscopic views are often poor in the acute setting, so this is often left until bleeding stops to allow more formal bowel prep. If bleeding is persistent it is still of value when attempting to distinguish which half of the colon is the source to allow planning of surgery (ie left or right hemicolectomy)
- ○ Mesenteric angiography – this does not have widespread availability as a specialist radiologist and an angiogram suite are required. Allows localisation of bleeding site and visualisation of angiodysplasia provided there is > 0.5 ml/min bleeding into the bowel lumen. If anatomy is favourable, the bleeding may be controlled by embolising the feeding vessel(s) at the same sitting. Use with caution in patients with renal impairment and type 2 diabetes mellitus due to the nephrotoxic nature of contrast agents.

Treatment

- Depends on underlying cause. Remember that although 80% of lower gastrointestinal bleeds stop spontaneously, severe bleeds can be life-threatening
- If patient is haemodynamically stable and not anaemic, then colonoscopy can be performed when the bleeding settles following formal bowel prep to optimise views
- Persistent bleeding requires both upper and lower gastrointestinal endoscopy
- If bleeding persists and the cause or site cannot be determined, a mesenteric angiogram is required (only if bleeding is active)
- If bleeding persists, laparotomy and bowel resection may be required if the source has been ascertained. If source is still unclear then a subtotal colectomy and end-ileostomy is needed. Persistent bleeding thereafter can be seen to arise from the stoma

Jaundice is generated by deposition of bilirubin, a breakdown product of haemoglobin, in the skin, sclerae and mucous membranes. Clinically jaundice is detectable when serum bilirubin is > 35 μmol/l. It is the most frequent mode of presentation of hepatic disease.

Jaundice may be divided into pre-hepatic (excess of unconjugated bilirubin that the liver cannot metabolise into conjugated bilirubin), hepatic (due to hepatocellular disease, consists of both unconjugated and conjugated bilirubin) and post-hepatic/obstructive (impairment of extra-hepatic biliary drainage – most common 'surgical' causes of jaundice) (Table 2.9). The causes of the three subtypes of jaundice are listed in Table 2.10.

Table 2.9 Classification of jaundice

	Pre-hepatic	**Hepatic**	**Obstructive**
Conjugated bilirubin	Normal	Normal	High
Urobilinogen	High	Normal	Nil

Table 2.10 Causes of jaundice

Pre-hepatic	**Hepatic**	**Obstructive**
Hereditary spherocytosis Rhesus incompatibility Incompatible blood transfusion Haemolysis Congestive cardiac failure	Infective hepatitis Liver tumour (primary or secondary) Cirrhosis Gilbert's syndrome Primary biliary cirrhosis Wilson's disease Cystic fibrosis α_1-Antitrypsin deficiency Drug induced	Common bile duct stones Bile duct strictures (eg from previous surgery) Extrinsic compression by tumour (eg head of pancreas tumour) Mirizzi's syndrome Cholangiocarcinoma

History

Clinical assessment and investigations are aimed at determining the cause to guide management.

Important questions to ask:

- Pale stool (reduced stercobilinogen) and dark urine (increased conjugated bilirubin) suggest obstructive jaundice
- Pruritus? → obstructive
- Previous history of gallstones/right upper quadrant abdominal pain?
- Alcohol intake? → alcoholic hepatitis
- Travel, intravenous drug use, previous hepatitis exposure, joint pain, anorexia? → infective hepatitis
- Weight loss, constitutional symptoms, altered bowel habit, epigastric/back pain? → possible malignancy
- Jaundice since childhood? Family history? → haemolytic cause/enzyme deficiency
- Fevers? → associated with pre-hepatic conditions, cholangitis

---

REMEMBER CHARCOT'S TRIAD

Right upper quadrant abdominal pain + jaundice + fever/chills = bacterial cholangitis

---

Examination

Is a dilated gallbladder palpable? If so note importance of Courvoisier's law.

COURVOISIER'S LAW

An **enlarged**, **non-tender** gallbladder in the presence of **jaundice** is unlikely to be due to gallstones.

In this circumstance, carcinoma of the pancreas or extra-hepatic biliary tree is more likely. This is because gallstones are formed over a longer period of time, and this results in a shrunken, fibrotic gallbladder which does not distend easily. Conversely, a gallbladder containing stones is usually chronically fibrosed and incapable of enlargement.

- A lumpy, irregular hepatomegaly suggests malignant disease
- Stigmata of chronic liver disease (spider naevi, clubbing, ascites, palmar erythema) suggest hepatitis or cirrhosis
- Check left supraclavicular Virchow's node → metastatic upper gastrointestinal tumour

Investigations

Liver function tests

- Bilirubin > 35 μmol/l is compatible with clinical finding of jaundice
- High alkaline phosphatase with normal or moderately raised aspartate aminotransferase (AST)/alanine aminotransferase (ALT), high γ-glutamyl transferase (GGT) → obstructive
- High AST and ALT with normal or mildly raised alkaline phosphatase → hepatitic

Clotting

- Vitamin K is fat soluble, so will not be absorbed in obstructive jaundice
- Prothrombin time (PT)/INR normal in pre-hepatic jaundice
- PT/INR raised (and correctable with iv vitamin K) in post-hepatic jaundice

Urinalysis

- Raised urobilinogen suggests pre-hepatic or hepatic (as conjugated bilirubin is excreted into duodenum and converted to urobilinogen in ileum)
- No or reduced urobilinogen suggests obstructive (no conjugated bilirubin excreted into intestine)
- Raised bilirubin suggests obstructive jaundice

Ultrasound

Gold standard for identifying gallstones and measuring common bile duct. Note: The diameter of the common bile duct increases with age, although it should be considered pathological if it is measured above 8 mm in a patient < 70 years with extra-hepatic biliary obstruction (eg common bile duct stone). USS also accurately detects hepatic pathology. Views of the pancreas are often poor (seen better with CT).

Endoscopic retrograde cholangiopancreatography (ERCP)

- Used where there is evidence of common bile duct obstruction (ie common bile duct diameter > 8 mm)
- Defines ductal anatomy
- Identifies nature of obstruction
- Identifies level of obstruction
- Therapeutic – can be used for sphincterotomy, stone extraction, stenting and dilatation of strictures

ERCP is used selectively due to the associated risks – pancreatitis (3%), septicaemia, bleeding, perforation and death (< 1%).

Magnetic resonance cholangiopancreatography (MRCP)

- Allows clear imaging of extra-hepatic biliary tree
- Advantage over ERCP is that it is safe, although it does not allow therapeutic manoeuvres

---

COMPLICATIONS OF OPERATING ON JAUNDICED PATIENTS

- Bleeding (clotting dysfunction)
- Impaired wound healing
- Renal failure (hepato-renal syndrome)
- Peptic stress ulceration

GALLSTONE DISEASE

Gallstones are present in 10% of the population, of which only 20% will develop symptoms. Thus, cholecystectomy is reserved only for patients with symptomatic cholelithiasis.

USS is the radiological investigation of choice to establish a diagnosis and assess common bile duct diameter; a common bile duct diameter of > 8 mm suggest obstruction. This is most commonly because of migration of a gallstone into the common bile duct.

Of gallbladders removed at cholecystectomy, 2–4% have co-existing missed common bile duct stones. Elevated bilirubin, alkaline phosphatase or GGT suggest biliary obstruction. In this circumstance, an ERCP is necessary. ERCP acts as both a diagnostic modality to visualise the extra-hepatic bile ducts and a therapeutic tool to retrieve common bile duct stones and stent stenotic lesions.

COMPLICATIONS OF GALLSTONES

- Biliary colic
- Acute cholecystitis
- Chronic cholecystitis
- Empyema
- Mucocele
- Carcinoma
- Perforation
- Cholangitis
- Pancreatitis
- Cholecystoduodenal fistula/gallstone ileus
- 'Porcelain' gallbladder
- Mirizzi's syndrome

COMPLICATIONS OF GALLSTONES

BILIARY COLIC

Arises from impaction of a gallstone in Hartmann's pouch resulting in rapid-onset, painful gallbladder contractions, which persist until the stone becomes dislodged.

History

Severe episodic right upper quadrant and epigastric pain referred to the right shoulder and exacerbated by fatty food. Rapid onset, lasting 2–4 hours.

Examination

- No peritonism overlying gallbladder
- Afebrile

Investigations

- WCC, LFT and amylase normal
- USS to establish diagnosis

Treatment

Analgesia and where appropriate elective cholecystectomy.

ACUTE CHOLECYSTITIS

Similar pathogenesis to biliary colic, but with the presence of infection. Thus, presentation differs from biliary colic due to presence of inflammation.

COMPLICATIONS OF ACUTE CHOLECYSTITIS

- Empyema
- Gallbladder perforation
- Choledocholithiasis (common bile duct stone)
- Cholecystenteric fistula/gallstone ileus
- Mirizzi's syndrome (gallstone lodged in either the cystic duct or the Hartmann's pouch causing external compression of the common hepatic duct, resulting in symptoms of obstructive jaundice)

Organisms associated with biliary infection may be Gram-negative (*E. coli*, *Klebsiella*, *Pseudomonas*, *Enterobacter*, *Proteus*) or Gram-positive (enterococci). Gram-negative infections can usually be treated using trimethoprim, ciprofloxacin or cephalosporins.

History

- Severe episodic right upper quadrant and epigastric pain referred to the right shoulder exacerbated by fatty food
- Associated fever, nausea and vomiting
- Symptoms typically start to improve by the second day and disappear by a week; persistence of symptoms and sepsis suggest abscess formation (empyema)

Examination

- Febrile and tachycardia
- Tenderness and peritonism over gallbladder
- May have positive **Murphy's sign** (pain with gentle pressure over the gallbladder during inspiration)

Investigations

- WCC
- LFT and amylase
- USS to establish diagnosis during admission

Treatment

- Initial management – analgesia, antibiotics (eg ciprofloxacin)
- Later – elective cholecystectomy or percutaneous drainage of empyema in elderly or surgically unfit patients

CHRONIC CHOLECYSTITIS

Repeated attacks of acute inflammation make the gallbladder scarred, shrunken and thick walled. The ability to concentrate and store bile diminishes. The gallbladder generally contains sludge or gallstones that often obstruct the cystic duct.

History

- Recurrent right upper quadrant and epigastric pain referred to the right shoulder exacerbated by fatty food
- Jaundice suggests common bile duct stone

Examination

- Tenderness over gallbladder

Treatment

- Analgesia
- Plan for elective cholecystectomy

COMMON BILE DUCT STONES (CHOLEDOCHOLITHIASIS)

History

Signs that suggest common bile duct stones includes dark urine, jaundice and pancreatitis. These may be complicated by infection of the biliary tract (ascending cholangitis)

Examination

Pyrexia, fever, rigors and sweats suggest superadded sepsis (cholangitis).

Investigations

- ↑ Alkaline phosphatase and bilirubin
- USS shows dilated common bile duct with gallstones
- INR may be raised due to non-absorbance of vitamin K

Treatment

- ERCP is useful to distinguish from malignant bile duct obstruction. It can be used to retrieve stone prior to cholecystectomy
- Correct clotting with iv vitamin K
- Prophylactic antibiotics

ASCENDING CHOLANGITIS

Arises from biliary stasis within the common bile duct with superadded infection.

History

Classic presentation is known as Charcot's triad:

- Right upper quadrant abdominal pain
- Jaundice
- Fever/chills

Examination

- Tenderness over gallbladder
- Jaundice
- Pyrexia

Investigations

- ↑ Alkaline phosphatase, GGT and bilirubin
- ↑ WCC
- INR may be raised due to non-absorbance of vitamin K

Treatment

- Intravenous fluids, nil by mouth
- Urinary catheter
- Correct clotting with iv vitamin K
- Intravenous antibiotics (eg ciprofloxacin + metronidazole or piperacillin)
- Urgent ERCP to demonstrate common bile duct obstruction and therapeutic sphincterotomy and stone retrieval. Less commonly, percutaneous trans-hepatic cholangiography (PTC) and drainage can be used for diagnostic purposes and draining infected bile

GALLSTONE PANCREATITIS

See Pancreatitis below.

PANCREATITIS

Pancreatitis is classified as being either mild or severe (Atlanta criteria, 1992) and either acute or chronic. Severe pancreatitis implies the presence of organ failure, local complications, or pancreatic necrosis. Such complications of pancreatitis are absent in its mild form.

The initial assessment and resuscitation of patients with acute pancreatitis cannot be compromised: 20% of cases are severe with up to 20% mortality. There may be hypoxia, dehydration, renal impairment and evidence of developing multiorgan failure. The principles of initial assessment and resuscitation are:

- Establish diagnosis and possible cause
- Distinguish between mild and severe
- Rehydrate
- Oxygenate
- Monitor
- Early organisation of HDU/ITU bed if severe attack

The two most common causes are gallstones in the common bile duct causing blockage of the pancreatic duct and alcohol excess. In children trauma and viral infection are recognised causes. The final pathway in the pathogenesis of pancreatitis is the premature activation of digestive enzymes within the acinar cells. Other causes are remembered by the mnemonic 'I GET SMASHED'.

CAUSES OF PANCREATITIS – I GET SMASHED

- **I**diopathic
- **G**allstones
- **E**thanol
- **T**rauma
- **S**teroids
- **M**umps (paramyxovirus) – also other viruses, eg Epstein–Barr, cytomegalovirus
- **A**utoimmune (polyarteritis nodosa)
- **S**corpion/**s**nake bites – rare!
- **H**yperlipidaemia/hypocalcaemia/hypothermia
- **E**RCP – up to 5% risk, 1% risk of severe pancreatitis
- **D**rugs (azathioprine, thiazide diuretics)

IMPORTANT DIFFERENTIAL DIAGNOSES TO EXCLUDE

- Perforated duodenal ulcer
- Acute gastritis/peptic ulcer
- Acute cholecystitis
- Myocardial infarction
- Mesenteric ischaemia
- Rupture abdominal aortic aneurysm

History

- Upper abdominal pain commonly radiates to back
- Nausea and vomiting
- Symptoms associated with underlying aetiology (eg jaundice, dark urine for common bile duct stone)

Examination

- Hypoxia – check respiratory rate, oxygen saturation, chest auscultation
- Shock – check pulse, BP
- Dehydration – check mucous membranes, skin turgor and urine output
- Abdominal examination

  - Epigastric tenderness
  - Make sure no aneurysm present
  - **Cullen's sign** – periumbilical pigmentation
  - **Grey Turner's sign** – bilateral flank discoloration

- Biliary obstruction – check for jaundice
- Sepsis (eg from cholangitis) – check temperature

Investigations

Early investigations

- Amylase – rise not proportional to severity

  NOTE: lesser rises in serum amylase occur with perforated peptic ulcer or small bowel, mesenteric infarction, acute liver failure, cholangitis, renal failure and diabetic ketoacidosis. In addition, pregnancy generates an amylaemia which is not related to pancreatitis.

- eCXR – exclude pneumoperitoneum, pleural effusions
- AXR – not essential, but may show central small bowel distension ('sentinel loop' created by localised ileus)
- Raised bilirubin and/or alkaline phosphatase suggests common bile duct stone
- Electrocardiogram (ECG)

Do ALL the following investigations to calculate severity score:

- FBC
- U&E
- LFT
- Blood gas on air
- Glucose
- Calcium

- Age > 55 years
- WCC > 15×10^9/l
- Glucose > 11 mmol/l
- AST > 200 mmol/l
- Lactase dehydrogenase > 600 IU/l
- pO_2 < 8 kPa
- Albumin < 32 g/l
- Ca^{2+} < 2 mmol/l
- Urea > 16 mmol

Severe pancreatitis is predicted by three or more and requires HDU/ITU admission

Other scoring systems, eg APACHE II and Ransom, are equally valid

Subsequent investigations

- Daily serial CRP – monitor course of inflammatory process
- Daily assessment of U&E, WCC, Ca^{2+} and LFT until clinical improvement
- Request USS – to look for gallstones/dilated common bile duct
- CT with iv contrast – not routinely indicated during first 48 hours. Used in severe/non-resolving pancreatitis to detect local complications such as necrosis
- ERCP – controversial

Treatment

Mild pancreatitis

- Can be treated on main ward
- Oxygen
- iv fluids
- Urinary catheter – hourly output to be maintained > 50 ml/h
- Nil by mouth and nasogastric tube if vomiting
- Opioid analgesia
- DVT prophylaxis

Severe pancreatitis

- Transfer to HDU or ITU – senior involvement
- Hypoxia may require continuous positive airways pressure (CPAP) or intubation in the presence of acute respiratory distress syndrome (ARDS)
- Urinary catheter monitoring
- Central line and central venous pressure (CVP) monitoring
- Arterial line if blood gas derangement
- RRT if necessary

COMPLICATIONS OF PANCREATITIS

Local

- Pancreatic necrosis
- Pseudocyst
- Abscess

Systemic

- ARDS
- Acute renal failure
- Disseminated intravascular coagulation (DIC)
- Diabetes
- Relapse
- Chronicity

ABSCESSES

An abscess is collection of pus within the soft tissues. Pus consists of bacteria, acute inflammatory cells, protein exudate and necrotic tissue, and is surrounded by granulation tissue.

A WORD OF WARNING: GROIN ABSCESSES IN IV DRUG MISUSERS

NEVER incise and drain a groin abscess in an iv drug misuser without a prior USS. Injection into a femoral vessel is common and can create a false aneurysm with surrounding infection. Incision of this will result in life-threatening haemorrhage

History

The only evidence of deep abscesses may be the symptoms:

- Swinging fever, sweats, rigors
- Local pain
- Malaise
- Local effects, eg diarrhoea with a pelvic collection, seizure with cerebral abscess
- Injection site, history of foreign body

Examination

The four cardinal features of inflammation easily identify superficial abscesses:

- Calor (heat)
- Rubor (red)
- Dolor (pain)
- Tumour (swelling)

There is often a spot where the abscess is 'pointing', ie close to discharging to the surface.

Check for systemic sepsis:

- Flushed
- Pyrexia
- Dehydration – tachycardia, reduced urine output, dry tongue

Investigations

- Blood glucose
- FBC if septic
- U&E if appears dehydrated
- USS if abscess is an injection site in femoral triangle (see box on page 87) – will identify true abscess or false aneurysm with overlying infection

Treatment

The treatment is surgical drainage as antibiotic penetration into the abscess cavity is poor. The cavity is dressed (eg using alginate) to leave the wound edges open and facilitate discharge. Packs are changed daily. Prolonged antibiotic use is unadvised as the abscess will become hardened and develop a chronic infection ('antibioma'). Unless the abscess is superficial and small (< 3 cm) this should be done under GA for the patient's comfort and to allow sufficient de-roofing and washout. Hidden, deep cavities may be treated using USS/CT-guided drainage.

Drainage of superficial abscesses is straightforward and a good introduction to the operating theatre for the foundation doctor! Drainage of a superficial abscess is as follows:

- Clean and prep the overlying skin
- Palpate abscess and locate site of maximal fluctuance
- Incise the cavity over the most fluctuant part so that pus flows out. Extend the incision in two directions to form a cruciate incision
- Send pus for microbiological examination
- Break down loculi manually and excise necrotic tissue
- Wash out cavity with saline
- A dressing (eg alginate) should be inserted into the wound
- Change pack in 24 hours

Antibiotics only have a role if the patient is systemically unwell, septic or if there is a large area of surrounding erythema.

COMMON TYPES OF ABSCESS

Cutaneous

Staphylococcus aureus is the most common causative organism, although bowel commensal organisms become more common in abscesses nearer the perineum. These may occur due to a breach in the skin, infection of a sebaceous cyst or following a chronic skin infection. Treatment entails open incision and drainage and cavity packing.

Abscess formation in wounds following surgery is unfortunately common, particularly following emergency abdominal surgery. Superficial wound abscesses display the four cardinal features described above and can be easily recognised. Treatment involves opening the wound at that point to allow wound discharge.

Perianal

May be described as:

- Ischiorectal
- Perianal
- Intersphincteric
- Supralevator

Bowel organisms are most common causative organisms. Note that perianal abscesses may on occasions arise as a result of long-standing Crohn's disease or a malignancy. Treatment is incision and drainage following rigid sigmoidoscopy and examination under anaesthetic to exclude a fistula or rectal pathology. A biopsy of the rectum may be done to examine for Crohn's granulomas.

Pelvic

Pelvic abscesses are associated with swinging pyrexia, evidence of sepsis and altered bowel habit (diarrhoea). This may be secondary to another pathology (eg appendicitis, diverticulitis) or a complication of surgery. The cavity may be felt through the rectum and may thus be drained transrectally. Alternatively a CT-guided drain may be placed.

Deep pelvic/intraperitoneal abscesses can arise from diverticular disease, localised bowel perforation (eg eroding malignancy), intraoperative bowel spillage or anastomotic leakage.

Subphrenic

Subphrenic abscesses are associated with swinging pyrexia, evidence of sepsis, reduced bowel transit and upper abdominal pain radiating to the shoulder. Treatment involves CT/USS-guided percutaneous drainage or surgical washout.

Postoperative intra-abdominal abscess

This can complicate any laparotomy, particularly for local sepsis or bowel resection. Diagnosis can be difficult, but the presence of the following provides clues to the presence of an abdominal collection:

- ↑ Temperature – swinging
- ↑ WCC/CRP
- Persisting abdominal pain
- Non-resolving ileus after 5 days
- Diarrhoea

- Nausea and vomiting
- Bowel distension
- Anorexia

Mainstay of diagnosis is USS or CT. Treatment most commonly consists of radiologically guided percutaneous drainage or open surgical washout. Intravenous fluids and antibiotics will be required.

NECROTISING FASCIITIS

Necrotising fasciitis is a serious condition requiring prompt surgical attention. It is a rapidly progressing infection that spreads along fascial planes. It may follow surgery, bowel spillage or even a skin puncture. The infection causes thrombosis and tissue necrosis. The patient is systemically septic and there is often resultant multiorgan failure if intervention is delayed. Necrotising fasciitis of the scrotum is called **Fournier's gangrene**.

Necrotising fasciitis is usually caused by several organisms. The most commonly implicated are β-haemolytic streptococcus plus:

- Coliforms
- Anaerobes – including *Clostridium perfringens*
- Staphylococcus

History

- History of recent trauma or surgery
- Check for antibiotic allergy
- Predisposing factors: diabetes mellitus, steroid use, immunocompromise, malignancy

Examination

Skin

- Erythema
- Oedema
- Heat
- Necrosis
- Pus discharge
- Crepitus (gas in subcutaneous tissue)

General
- Pain
- Febrile
- Tachycardia
- Dehydration

Investigations
- WCC, U&E, clotting, CRP
- ABG – look for acidosis
- Blood culture and pus swab – urgent Gram staining
- X-ray may show surgical emphysema (gas in subcutaneous tissue)
- CXR – at risk of ARDS

Treatment
- 100% oxygen and fluid resuscitation
- Analgesia
- Urinary catheter – monitor hourly output and strictly monitor fluid balance
- HDU/ITU input may be required if haemodynamically unstable or evidence of ARDS/organ failure
- Intravenous infusion to maintain hydration
- Intravenous broad-spectrum antibiotics including anaerobic cover

URGENT surgical debridement is needed for any chance of survival. All infected and non-viable tissue must be aggressively debrided. There is often surprisingly extensive involvement of subcutaneous fat. The infected area is debrided up to healthy tissue, and packed. The wound is inspected initially daily to remove further necrotic tissue and change the dressing.

PAINFUL ANORECTAL CONDITIONS

ANORECTAL SEPSIS

The anal canal is a 3–4 cm epithelium-lined muscular tube, consisting of the internal sphincter (thickening of circular muscle) and the somatic external sphincter. The anal glands lie in the intersphincteric space and their ducts drain into the anus at the dentate line.

Abscesses start as infection in the anal glands and can track in different directions:

- If pus remains in the intersphincteric space, it forms an **intersphincteric abscess**
- Drainage inferiorly through the intersphincteric space leads to **perianal abscess** if pus collects subcutaneously, or an **intersphincteric fistula** if it discharges through the skin
- Drainage laterally through external sphincters leads to an **ischiorectal abscess**
- Drainage medially forms a **submucous abscess**

Over a third of anorectal abscesses are recurrent.

History

The abscess is usually characterised by a hot, painful lump in the perianal or buttock region. The history is usually short. Recurrent painful swellings or a long history may suggest a fistula-in-ano. There may be pus discharge, fever and chills.

Check for:

- History/symptoms suggestive of Crohn's disease
- Previous anal surgery
- Diabetes

Examination

- The classic signs of acute examination. Rubor, calor, dolor and tumour (described in Abscesses, pages 87–91)
- Look for pus discharge, which would suggest a fistula
- General examination for signs of sepsis and dehydration
- Exclude differential diagnoses: anal carcinoma, lymphoma and hidradenitis suppurativa
- Important not to miss Fournier's gangrene

Investigations

Usually no investigation is required for simple abscess. The anatomy of complex fistulae, eg where there is a history of several operations, can be visualised by endoanal ultrasound or MRI.

Treatment

- Examine under anaesthesia – to identify an associated abscess
- Rigid sigmoidoscopy to exclude underlying disease
- Incision/de-roofing of abscess
- Pack cavity
- If patient is well and comfortable, can be discharged the following day

If a fistula is seen, a probe must be passed along it. If it is low (ie below the level of the sphincters), then the tract can be laid open. If a high fistula (above the level of the sphincters) is present, then a **Seton** suture can be used. This is a suture or plastic sling that is fed through the abscess and helps define the anatomy and allows a path for pus to drain. It can also be tightened in stages to allow healing without disruption to the sphincter complex and resulting incontinence.

GOODSALL'S LAW

Allows prediction of the path of a fistula if the external opening can be seen. Those with external openings in the posterior half of the perianal area usually have an internal opening in the posterior midline with the tract extending in a horse-shoe shape. Those with external openings in the anterior perineum, the internal opening will usually originate in the anterior quadrant of the anus, with the tract extending in a radial manner

FISSURE-IN-ANO

Breach in squamous epithelium of lower third of anus.

History

- Usually a short history of severe anal pain made worse during passage of stools
- There is usually a history of straining and passage of hard stools, causing the patient to fear defaecation
- Rectal bleeding is seen after defaecation, usually on wiping. The blood is bright red and not in stools

Examination

- Patient is usually in too much pain to allow digital examination
- The fissure is seen as a tear (approximately 1 cm), more common in the posterior midline (90%) although fissures can also be seen in anterior midline
- Sentinel skin tag overlying the fissure.
- Multiple fissures may be seen in Crohn's disease

Treatment

Non-surgical

- Lactulose
- Lidocaine gel
- 0.2% or 0.4% glyceryl trinitrate cream twice daily for 6 weeks (warn of associated headaches) or 2% diltiazem paste twice daily

Surgical

- Lateral sphincterotomy – warn of risk of sphincter injury. This is higher in multiparous women who may have pre-existing sphincter weakness (will need preoperative endoanal USS)
- Anal stretch no longer performed due to unacceptable risk of sphincter injury

PERIANAL HAEMATOMA

Presents with acute excruciating perianal pain, made worse with sitting and walking. A tense dark swelling is seen at the anal verge. Treatment is analgesia, ice pack and reassurance. Improvement is seen by 2–3 days. If the pain is unbearable, it may be evacuated under local or general anaesthetic.

THROMBOSED (STRANGULATED) HAEMORRHOID

History

- Painful haemorrhoids (usually long history of haemorrhoids)
- May be bleeding
- Painful defaecation

Examination

- Dark thrombosis within haemorrhoid.

Treatment

- Reassure patient – improvement usually seen after 2–3 days
- Cold compress
- Analgesia (NSAIDs effective provided not contraindicated in patient)
- Lactulose
- Surgical – emergency haemorrhoidectomy if conservative treatment fails

LUMPS AND BUMPS

The majority of skin lesions are benign.

History

- Duration of swelling
- Pain
- Change in size – is it growing?
- Does the lump disappear – herniae disappears on lying
- Causative events, eg trauma, heavy lifting may cause herniae
- Any other similar lumps elsewhere
- Systemic symptoms

Examination

- Site – describe in relation to fixed anatomical landmarks
- Shape
- Size
- Surface
- Consistency – hard, soft, fluctuant
- Composition – solid, fatty, air filled
- Compressibility/reducibility
- Tenderness

- Temperature
- Overlying inflammation
- Pulsatility
- Relation to surrounding structure – includes fixity to underlying muscle
- Examine regional lymph nodes

Does a general examination depending on findings, eg an enlarged lymph node requires its draining regions plus the remainder of the lymphoreticular system to be examined.

SKIN LESIONS

Table 2.11 Skin lesions – terms you should know

Macule	Flat circumscribed area demarcated by colour from surrounding tissue
Papule	Solid raised discrete lesion of 5 mm or less
Plaque	Flat but elevated area, usually greater than 5 mm
Nodule	Solid raised discrete lesion greater than 5 mm in greatest dimension
Blister	Non-specific term for fluid-filled lesion
Vesicle	Fluid-filled lesion of 5 mm or less
Cyst	Fluid collection in an endothelial- or epithelial-lined sac
Pustule	Small pus-filled elevated area of the skin with discrete borders
Excoriation	Lesion of traumatic nature with epidermal loss in a generally linear shape
Onycholysis	Loosening/loss of nail substance
Ulcer	Loss of epidermis and dermis

Sebaceous (epidermoid) cyst

Sebaceous cysts most often arise from swollen hair follicles. They contain keratin which appears as a cheesy white/grey material if cut. Sebaceous cysts may become infected to form an abscess.

History

- Non-tender lump under skin. May be slowly growing. Occasionally history of trauma to area
- If infected, there will be a short history of pain, redness and possibly a purulent discharge

Examination

- Most commonly found on head, truck and upper limb
- Well defined, variable size, round, rubbery firm, mobile to underlying tissue but not fixed to skin
- Usually a punctum is visible
- If infected, it will display the characteristics of an abscess (see pages 87–91).

Treatment

These are not dangerous and the patient can be reassured. Indication for excision under local anaesthetic are patient anxiety, symptoms (eg scalp lesion disturbing hair combing) or history of infection.

Acutely infected sebaceous cysts may be treated with anti-staphylococcal antibiotics and later excision. Abscesses will need formal drainage.

Lipoma

A lipoma is a benign tumour of the fat cells in a thin, fibrous capsule. They may arise anywhere, but are commonly seen on the torso, neck, proximal limbs and axillae. Liposarcoma, a rare separate entity, is a malignant growth and is characterised by more rapid growth and invasion. Dercum's disease is a rare inherited disorder characterised by multiple lipomas that can cause symptoms because of pressure on surrounding structures.

History

Painless and slow growing.

Examination

Well-defined, mobile, spherical, soft, non-tender, variable size and not fixed to skin (unlike sebaceous cyst).

Management

- Reassure patient
- Excision under anaesthetic needed only if patient anxious or it is causing symptoms

Seborrhoeic keratosis

Seborrhoeic keratosis is a common benign skin lesion found elderly people. It is derived from epidermal cells.

History

Usually asymptomatic, but there may be history of itching or bleeding.

Examination

- Raised papule of various brown pigmentation which can bleed if disturbed
- Appear as if 'stuck on' to the skin surface

Management

- Reassurance
- If symptomatic they can be burned or shaved off under local anaesthetic

Naevus

Naevi are benign melanotic lesions – some varieties carry a malignant potential. The importance of a naevus is to distinguish it from a melanoma. Benign naevi are asymptomatic and the patient usually presents due to concern or cosmetic issues. There is variability is terms of size, shape, colour and hair covering. Naevi require excision if there are any features suggestive of melanoma (see below). Three variations are described on the basis of their histological position within skin:

- **Intradermal** (most common) – may be light or dark, flat or raised. Hairy moles will be intradermal. Not found on the soles of the hands or feet
- **Junctional** (between the epidermis and dermis) – may occur anywhere. Has malignant potential
- **Compound** (intradermal and junctional features) – similar macroscopic appearance to intradermal but does have malignant potential

If signs of malignant change are present in a naevus, check local lymph nodes. Excision is recommended.

ABDOMINAL WALL HERNIAE

Remember the definition of a hernia:

> Abnormal protrusion of a viscus (or part of a viscus) through a defect in the wall of its containing cavity.

Abdominal wall herniae consist of a peritoneal sac, which may contain fat, bowel or rarely other structures such as bladder. The majority occur in the groin.

Herniae are described on clinical grounds as either reducible or irreducible. Irreducible herniae are further subclassified as:

- **Incarcerated** – irreducible but not obstructed and not ischaemic
- **Obstructed** – lumen of viscus occluded
- **Strangulated** – blood supply occluded leading to ischaemia and infarction

Obstructed herniae will cause symptoms and signs of intestinal obstruction (described on pages 53–59). Strangulated herniae cause bowel wall ischaemia, resulting in pain and physical manifestations of sepsis. Irreducible herniae require surgery. Incarcerated herniae presenting out of hours can be operated on the next day, but obstructed and strangulated types need to be dealt with urgently.

Table 2.12 Lumps and bumps – differential diagnosis

Skin/subcutaneous	Sebaceous cyst Lipoma
Hernia	Inguinal hernia Femoral hernia Obturator hernia
Haematological	Lymphadenopathy
Vascular	Saphena varix Iliac/femoral artery aneurysm
Gastrointestinal	Appendix mass/abscess Caecal carcinoma Ileitis Ileocaecal tuberculosis Psoas abscess/bursitis
Urological	Transplanted kidney (sited in iliac fossa) Ectopic testicle

AETIOLOGY OF ABDOMINAL WALL HERNIAE

- Trauma/previous surgery (incisional hernia)
- Nerve injury (eg ilioinguinal nerve injury following appendicectomy leading to right inguinal hernia)
- Loss of muscle strength (age)
- Widening of natural defect (eg hiatus hernia)
- Increased intra-abdominal pressure
- Straining
- Chronic cough
- Constipation
- Bladder outflow obstruction
- Pregnancy

History

- How long has the hernia been there?
- Previous surgery?
- Can the hernia be pushed back inside? If not – how long has this been for?
- Is the hernia painful? → persistent pain suggests strangulation
- Any vomiting/constipation/abdominal distension/colicky pain? → obstruction
- Past medical history and drug history?
- Employment – heavy labour predisposes to hernia development; postoperatively, there is a need to avoid heavy lifting for 2–4 weeks which may have ramifications for the patient

Examination

- Abdominal examination to confirm diagnosis and establish type of hernia
- Reducibility
- Scars from previous surgery
- Evidence of obstruction – abdominal distension, increased bowel sounds, dehydration
- Evidence of strangulation – hernia tenderness, erythema of overlying skin, pyrexia, tachycardia
- Full system examination to assess fitness for surgery

Common abdominal wall herniae

Inguinal

These are the most common type. Remember that indirect herniae (80%) pass through the deep inguinal ring ('midpoint of the inguinal ligament') and run within the spermatic cord towards the superficial inguinal ring (above and medial to pubic tubercle). A reduced indirect hernia can thus be controlled by point pressure over the deep ring. A direct hernia (20%) passes directly through the defect in the posterior wall of the inguinal canal (transversalis muscle) medial to the deep ring and inferior epigastric vessels. Direct herniae rarely strangulate, this is more common in the indirect type. Both types may be repaired by open surgery or laparoscopically.

Table 2.13 Contents of the inguinal canal

Artery to the vas	Ilioinguinal nerve	Vas/round ligament
Testicular artery	Genital nerve	Pampiniform plexus
Cremasteric artery	Sympathetic nerve	Lymphatics

Femoral

These pass through the femoral ring and are prone to incarceration, obstruction and strangulation. The femoral ring is defined anteriorly by the inguinal ligament, medially by the lacunar ligament, lateral the femoral vein and posteriorly the pectineal fascia.

The neck is tight and at high risk of strangulation and so femoral herniae are at high risk and need to be operated on urgently. During surgery to close the femoral ring, care must be taken not to accidentally compress the femoral vein. A Richter's hernia is where part of the intestinal circumference becomes trapped within the hernia which may become strangulated without luminal obstruction.

Paraumbilical/umbilical

Umbilical herniae (through the umbilicus) arise in childhood and only require repair if persistent after 2 years of age. This can be remembered by the **rule of 3s**:

- 3% of live births
- Operate at $\geq$ 3 years old (as most regress by 2 years)
- 0.3% need repair

Conversely, paraumbilical herniae (just above or below the umbilicus) are acquired through increased intra-abdominal pressure. The sac contains omentum or/and small bowel which may strangulate in 20% cases.

Epigastric

- Through the linea alba above the umbilicus
- The defect is often small, and the sac usually only contains fat but can cause significant pain

Incisional

This is a complication of about 10% of all abdominal incisions. There is commonly a history of postoperative wound infection. Other factors associated with incisional herniae include: poor surgical technique, excess tension along the suture line, malnutrition, diabetes, ischaemia, obesity, renal failure, steroid therapy and malignancy. Since the defect is often wide, strangulation is uncommon although the patient may have pain as well as cosmetic concerns. These may be treated by either primary sutured or mesh repair, by open or laparoscopic methods.

Other herniae

- Spigelian (lateral edge of rectus)
- Lumbar (through lumbar triangle)
- Obturator (through obturator canal – produces medial thigh pain)

STOMAS

Stomas are surgically created connections between internal organs and cavities and the skin. In the case of GI stomas, they are named depending on the part of intestine that has been brought to the skin. In general, they have three uses:

- Drainage
- Enteral feeding
- Diversion of faeces or urine

Small-bowel stomas are made in patients with intestinal perforation or ischaemia in whom an anastomosis is considered unsafe. Stomas may also be described as:

- End stoma – where the bowel is divided, and the proximal end brought through the abdominal wall
- Loop stoma – where a loop of bowel is brought to the skin still in continuity. These allow for fast surgery but may allow proximal bowel content to spill distally
- Feeding stoma

PLACEMENT

Whenever possible, an ileostomy or colostomy site along with an alternative site needs to be marked preoperatively by a dedicated stoma therapist. To allow stoma care, it should be:

- Distant from the incision
- Through the midportion of the rectus abdominis muscle
- Away from skin folds (eg, groin, flank), bony prominences (eg, rib cage, iliac spine) and umbilicus
- Compatible with the clothing worn by the patient

COMMON TYPES OF STOMA

Gastrostomy

Percutaneous tube located in epigastrium, placed by direct or endoscopic visualisation into stomach. Used for feeding or gastric decompression, eg PEG (percutaneous endoscopic gastrostomy) tube.

Jejunostomy

Tube placed percutaneously into jejunum to allow enteral feeding, eg following oesophagectomy to allow enteral feeding without placing strain on the proximal anastomosis.

Ileostomy

Terminal ileum brought to skin in the right iliac fossa either as an end or loop stoma used to divert faecal flow away from colon. Loop stomas have the ileum in continuity and are usually used as a temporary means of defunctioning a distal anastomosis or decompressing a distal obstruction. A 'bridge' is used to maintain shape and is removed after a week. An end stoma has the ileum in discontinuation and is used following either proctocolectomy or a right hemicolectomy where an ileocolic anastomosis has been judged too risky or impractical. An end ileostomy is obvious from its spout shape (fashioned to keep irritant small bowel effluent away from skin) and its position in the right iliac fossa. Produces a liquid effluent.

Colostomy

Any part of the colon may be exteriorised to the skin to decompress distal obstruction or because distal bowel has been resected and a low pelvic anastomosis is at risk of leaking. Usually found in left iliac fossa and is flush with skin. A colostomy, especially a distal one, produces solid stools.

A loop colostomy is used for decompression of a distal obstruction or to protect a distal anastomosis. An end colostomy is used following a major bowel resection where the anastomosis is at risk of leakage (eg Hartmann's procedure) or is not technically feasible (resection).

Mucous fistula

Distal end of transected colon brought to skin for decompression (remember that a fistula is a communication between two epithelialised surfaces – in this case skin of the abdominal wall and anus). The proximal end of bowel will also be brought out as either an end ileostomy or colostomy depending on the site of transection. Usually in left iliac fossa and is flush with skin. No faeces will be produced but epithelium-derived mucus may be seen.

Double-barrel stoma

An end stoma and mucous fistula that have been sited side by side. This position allows easy reversal (rejoining two ends together) at a later date.

Table 2.14 Differentiating stomas

Colostomy	Ileostomy
Left iliac fossa	Right iliac fossa
Produces faeces	Liquid effluent
Flush with skin	2- to 4-cm spout to protect skin
Permanent: abdomino-perineal resection	Permanent: panproctocolectomy
Temporary: Hartmann's operation	Temporary: defunctioning loop ileostomy (eg after anterior repair)

COMPLICATIONS OF STOMAS

Local

- Necrosis
- Detachment
- Retraction
- Stenosis
- Prolapse
- Ulceration and bleeding
- Parastomal herniation
- Fistula formation
- Leakage and skin irritation
- Granulomata and bleeding

Systemic

- Dehydration and salt depletion from excess stoma output
- Gallstones (if distal ileum resected – disturbed bile reabsorption)
- Odour and social difficulty

BREAST DISEASE

CAUSES OF BREAST LUMPS

Carcinoma

- Often painless
- Nipple retraction
- Skin dimpling, peau d'orange

Fibroadenoma ('breast mouse')

- 15–35 years
- 2–3 cm diameter
- Mobile
- Discrete
- Firm
- Non-tender

Continued over

CAUSES OF BREAST LUMPS (*continued*)

Phyllodes tumour

- Highly cellular type of fibroadenoma
- Can recur

Fibrocystic disease

- 20–45 years
- Changes with hormonal environment – cyclic breast pain
- Can be multiple
- Usually upper outer quadrant

Abscess

- From suppuration of acute mastitis – *S. aureus*
- Painful
- Tender
- Red
- Fluctuant

Fat necrosis

- Trauma and rupture of fat cells – may become calcified

Duct ectasia

- 50 years +
- Multiparous, smoker
- Dilatation of periareolar ducts
- Painful
- Nipple retraction due to fibrosis
- Creamy/green nipple discharge

Breast lumps are investigated by triple assessment:

- Clinical examination
- Radiological – mammography/breast USS
- Pathological – fine needle aspiration (FNA) and cytology/core biopsy

History

- Duration
- Pain
- Nipple discharge/bleeding
- Previous breast lump
- Menarche
- Menopause
- Obstetric/gynaecological history
- Breast feeding or OCP
- Family history

Examination

- Examine both breasts by quadrants
- Scars
- Lumps

  - Single or multiple
  - Skin tethering
  - Fixation to muscle
  - Overlying skin changes

- Nipple

  - Discharge
  - Inversion
  - Bleeding

- Lymph nodes

  - Axilla
  - Cervical
  - Mobile or fixed

- General examination looking for metastases – liver edge

Investigations

- USS if under 35 years
- Mammogram – cranio-caudal and oblique views
- FNA/punch biopsy/Tru-Cut biopsy

Treatment

Depends upon triple assessment diagnosis after appropriate counselling.

NIPPLE DISCHARGE

Nipple discharge may be caused by:

- Duct ectasia – green or brown discharge from one or more openings. Occurs in 40- to 50-year-olds. May be associated with nipple retraction due to surrounding mastitis. Treat by excision
- Duct papilloma – bleeding from nipple. Treat by excision
- Eczema of nipple – usually bilateral but may be confused with Paget's disease. Here, invasive ductal tumour invades cutaneous tissue. Send skin scrapings to differentiate

THYROID DISEASE

The thyroid consists of two lobes, and sometimes a pyramidal lobe, linked by an isthmus at the level of the second to fourth tracheal rings. The pretracheal fascia binds it to the trachea, allowing it to move with swallowing. Each lobe receives two arteries (superior thyroid from external carotid and inferior thyroid from subclavian via the thyrocervical trunk) and three veins (upper and middle thyroid vein draining to internal jugular and lower vein draining to the subclavian). Surgically important relations are the parathyroid glands and recurrent laryngeal nerves. The recurrent laryngeal nerves innervate the intrinsic muscles of the larynx and ascend from the vagus in the tracheo-oesophageal grooves where they lie in particularly close proximity to the inferior thyroid arteries. Injury causes ipsilateral vocal cord paralysis with voice hoarseness. The nearby superior laryngeal nerves have a lesser role in vocal cord control, although injury may cause alteration in pitch.

GOITRE

Examination

A goitre is any enlargement of the thyroid gland. In determining the cause, ask yourself whether the thyroid swelling is a solitary nodule, multinodular or diffuse.

- **Inspection**: From the front establish whether there is a swelling and whether this moves up with swallowing. Is the swelling in the midline, unilateral or either side of midline? Hoarse voice suggests recurrent laryngeal nerve compression

- **Palpate**: Is the trachea deviated in the suprasternal notch? Standing from behind with patient looking forward and neck slightly flexed, feel both sides of gland with the flat of the finger tips. If a swelling is palpable, is it: single or multiple nodules or a diffuse enlargement? Does it move with swallowing? Feel for lymphadenopathy along deep cervical chain
- **Percuss**: Sternum to determine retrosternal descent
- **Auscultate**: Vascular thyrotoxic glands may be associated with a bruit
- Proceed to examine for thyroid status

Table 2.15 Causes of goitre

Solitary nodule	Euthyroid	Cyst Adenoma Malignancy Amyloidosis
	Hyperthyroid	Functioning adenoma
Multinodular	Euthyroid	Multinodular goitre
	Hyperthyroid	Multinodular goitre with dominant functioning adenoma Toxic nodular goitre
Diffuse	Euthyroid	Hyperplastic Autoimmune thyroiditis Inflammatory thyroiditis
	Hyperthyroid	Graves' disease

Investigations

- Thyroid function tests (TFTs)
- USS – establishes size and whether lesions are single or multiple and cystic or solid. Note that although most solid lesions are benign, USS cannot distinguish between benign and malignant nodules. A malignant neoplasm may be incorporated in the wall of a cystic nodule
- Fine needle aspiration (FNA) – safe procedure which should be performed on all thyroid nodules. Distinguishes between solid and cystic disease. FNA may distinguish between benign and malignant pathologies with the *exception of follicular neoplasms*, where differentiation between adenoma and carcinoma is not possible

Routine investigation of goitre include TFT, USS and FNA. Assessment may also include:

- Radioisotope scan (^{31}I, ^{123}I or ^{99}Tch) – functional assessment of gland. 'Cold' areas are non-functioning areas and 'hot' areas are toxic. Cannot distinguish between benign and malignant lesions. About 10–15% cold nodules are malignant. Hot nodules are invariably benign
- CT scan – accurately determines size, extent, retrosternal extension and nodularity of gland. Also may establish local lymphadenopathy

THYROID NEOPLASIA

Benign

- Follicular adenoma – most common benign tumour, usually > 2 cm diameter. Cannot be distinguished from malignancy by FNA as capsule invasion is differentiating factor. All follicular lesions identified with FNA need excision
- Papillary adenoma – rare but requires excision due to potential for malignant transformation
- Toxic adenoma – uncommon, representing 5% of solitary nodules. Diagnosis established with isotope scan. Requires excision

Malignant

- Papillary carcinoma (60%) – most common malignancy. Peak 30–40 years. Slow growing. Fifty per cent are multifocal. Lymph node metastases are common, needing lymph node dissection. Unencapsulated. Often thyroid stimulating hormone (TSH) dependent so postoperative thyroxine to depress TSH can improve survival
- Follicular carcinoma (20%) – peak 40–60 years. Unifocal. Blood-borne metastases to lung, brain and bone. Encapsulated, and 20% of follicular lesions found with FNA are malignant. Frozen section histological analysis during surgery can confirm diagnosis. Radio-iodine scanning can detect metastases or recurrence
- Medullary (5%) – any age. Mode of spread – lymph. Associated with multiple endocrine neoplasia (MEN) syndrome 2, with 20% familial. Secretes calcitonin and CEA, with serum calcitonin measured to determine recurrence or metastasis following resection

- Anaplastic (5%). Occurs in elderly people and is associated with rapid growth. Local invasion may result in recurrent laryngeal nerve palsy and tracheal compression, early lymphatic spread and blood-borne metastasis to lung, bone and brain
- Lymphoma (5%). Increased risk with Hashimoto's thyroiditis

INDICATIONS FOR THYROIDECTOMY

- Established or suspected neoplasia
- Toxic nodule/goitre
- Tracheal compression
- Cosmesis

Table 2.16 Complications of thyroidectomy

Haemorrhage	Can cause tracheal obstruction and death. If there is a concern about postoperative bleeding then senior review must be sought ASAP. If there is evidence of airway obstruction, all layers of the wound need to be opened to decompress the haematoma. Suture cutters/clip removers should be available by the patient's bed
Recurrent laryngeal nerve injury	May be permanent or temporary. Permanent bilateral nerve injury requires tracheostomy or laser arytenoidectomy. Preoperative cord inspection is essential
Superior laryngeal nerve injury	Alteration in voice pitch. No specific treatment but professionals that rely on their voice must be counselled
Hypocalcaemia Thyrotoxic crisis Hypothyroidism Pneumothorax Wound complications	

THYROTOXICOSIS

Overproduction of T_3 and T_4 may occur due to:

- Graves' disease
- Toxic multinodular goitre
- Toxic adenoma

History

- Anxious and irritable
- Hot and sweaty
- Reduced weight but increased appetite
- Diarrhoea
- Oligomenorrhoea

Examination

- Tachycardia at rest or atrial fibrillation
- Fine tremor
- Exophthalmos
- Lid lag
- Pretibial myxoedema
- Carotid bruit

Investigations

- $\uparrow T_3, T_4$
- $\downarrow$ TSH
- ECG may show atrial fibrillation or tachycardia

Treatment

Non-operative

- Carbimazole – avoid in pregnancy
- Radioactive iodine – 10% get recurrence

Surgery

- Graves' disease and toxic multinodular goitre – subtotal thyroidectomy
- Toxic adenoma – lobectomy

CHAPTER 3

VASCULAR SURGERY

J GHOSH AND M G WALKER

TOPICS

PERIPHERAL ARTERIAL DISEASE

Peripheral arterial disease is predominantly secondary to atherosclerosis. It affects 5% of men > 50 years and has an increasing incidence with age in both sexes. Although this can occur anywhere in the arterial tree, the lower limbs are most affected. The two most commonly affected sites are the distal superficial femoral artery at the adductor hiatus and at the bifurcation of the common femoral artery within the femoral triangle.

Atherosclerosis is a slowly progressing disease with symptoms developing gradually over time. Importantly, this gradual pathogenesis allows time for development of a collateral circulation that provides an alternative route for blood to travel. Thus, even a slowly developing proximal occlusion may still allow blood to reach the distal extremities.

The principal symptom of chronic lower limb arterial insufficiency is **intermittent claudication** (Latin *claudicare* – to limp). Intermittent claudication is a **cramping** pain felt in muscle groups that is:

- Produced by physical exertion
- Made worse when walking uphill
- Relieved by rest

Intermittent claudication occurs at a constant walking distance and is predictably relieved by a duration of rest. Lower limb claudication is often described anatomically on the basis of the location of the prominent atherosclerotic disease: aorto-iliac, femoro-popliteal and 'distal' (ie distal to the popliteal artery) disease.

Critical ischaemia occurs when blood flow falls below a minimal level required to maintain limb viability. Symptoms appear while at rest ('rest pain') and tissue loss (ulceration) may be seen. Rest pain is a **burning** pain in the distal foot, often worse at night when the foot is elevated, and relieved by placing the leg in a dependent position.

Peripheral bypass surgery is reserved for individuals with debilitating short distance claudication or with critical limb ischaemia. These patients will require angiography with a view to planning arterial bypass surgery/angioplasty if possible.

History

- Claudication distance. This should not vary on flat ground, but is worse uphill. Pain due to intervertebral disc prolapse is worse walking downhill ('neurological' claudication)

- The muscle group affected gives an indication of where the lesion is in the peripheral arterial tree. Femoro-popliteal disease results in calf pain. Aortic-iliac disease usually manifests as thigh/buttock pain but can also cause calf pain
- **Leriche's syndrome** is characterised by buttock intermittent claudication, sexual impotence and absent femoral pulses. It indicates bilateral aorto-iliac occlusion
- Patients with rest pain find it worse at night and experience relief after hanging their limb over the end of the bed
- Duration of symptoms
- Presence of risk factors for atherosclerotic disease
- Other cardiovascular symptoms:

  - Myocardial infarction/angina
  - Previous transient ischaemic attack (TIA)/stroke/amaurosis fugax
  - Hypertension

- Home circumstances and quality of life

RISK FACTORS FOR ATHEROSCLEROSIS

- Smoking
- Hypertension
- Diabetes mellitus
- Hyperlipidaemia
- Family history
- Male sex
- Homocystinaemia

Examination

- Note pulse, any evidence of atrial fibrillation, BP, clinical signs of anaemia, dehydration or sepsis
- Colour of limb – pale or mottled?
- Ulcers? check pressure areas and for surrounding infection
- Gangrene
- Check for infection between toes
- Assess temperature difference between limbs
- Palpate and record all pulses in limbs; record this by comparing pulses on both sides

- Palpate for abdominal aortic, femoral or popliteal aneurysm
- Capillary refill at hallux – press pulp of hallux for 5 seconds and count time for colour to refill: normal is < 3 seconds
- Auscultation over major arteries for bruits

Buerger's angle: With the patient lying supine, slowly elevate the straightened leg and see if the foot becomes white. The angle at which this happens is Buerger's angle. In health, the leg should be able to be elevated to 90°.

Buerger's sign: When a leg that has been elevated to demonstrate Buerger's angle is put in a dependent position, a positive sign is when the limb 'blushes'; implies severe ischaemia.

Hand-held Doppler: Listen over peripheral pulses. A signal may be heard even where a pulse is impalpable. In expert hands, the signal can be described as triphasic (normal), biphasic (moderate impairment to flow) or monophasic (significant flow disturbance). An absent signal indicates occlusion.

Ankle–brachial pressure index (ABPI) (Table 3.1): This is assessed using a hand-held Doppler, jelly to reduce acoustic impedance and a manual sphygmomanometer.

- The BP in both arms is recorded to make sure that there is no disparity suggesting subclavian artery stenosis. If there is, use the arm with the highest pressure
- Find the brachial artery with the hand-held Doppler – this is most superficial just medial to the biceps tendon. The sphygmomanometer cuff is placed around the biceps and inflated until the Doppler signal disappears. Slowly reduce the cuff pressure until the signal reappears and document this reading
- Repeat this placing the cuff around the cuff around the thigh and Doppler over either the dorsalis pedis or posterior tibial artery, whichever gives the strongest signal. Calculate the ratio of the two pressure values

Table 3.1 Ankle–brachial pressure index

0.9–1.2	Normal
0.4–0.8	Moderate arterial disease Consistent with claudication
< 0.4	Severe ischaemia Consistent with development of rest pain

Investigations

- FBC, U&E, cholesterol, clotting, glucose
- CXR
- ECG
- **Arterial ultrasound scan with duplex** – determines degree of blood flow down limb and sites of arterial stenosis or occlusion. The waveform of the Doppler signal, described as triphasic (normal), biphasic (moderate disease) or monophasic (significant disease), will also give an indication of severity of disease
- **Angiography** (intra-arterial contrast, CT or magnetic resonance) – provides gold standard anatomical definition of the arterial tree. This is only done when surgery or angioplasty/stent is being considered. The risks of intra-arterial angiography are: bleeding, false aneurysm, thrombosis and distal embolisation and allergic reaction to contrast. Also, note that contrast medium can cause nephrotoxicity, and use in patients with renal impairment must be carefully considered. Patients with type 2 diabetes should stop metformin for 48 hours due to the risk of lactic acidosis

DIFFERENTIAL DIAGNOSIS OF LIMB PAIN

- Peripheral vascular disease
- Muscular pain
- Arthritis
- DVT
- Cellulitis
- Osteomyelitis
- Varicose veins
- Spinal stenosis (neuropathic claudication)
- Compartment syndrome
- Myositis

Treatment

This may involve medical, interventional radiology and bypass graft surgery alone or in combination.

Atherosclerosis is multifocal disease and these patients frequently have co-morbidities. Management of risk factors such as smoking, hypertension, hypercholesterolaemia and diabetes is the most important intervention for reducing the impact of atherosclerotic disease. There is often coronary artery disease and a cardiology opinion is required if there is a history of cardiac symptoms. Patients should be on life-long antiplatelet medication and a statin unless contraindicated. Weight loss should be advised in overweight patients.

Patients with stable claudication will be treated in most centres by medical risk reduction and entry to a supervised exercise programme. This may be in conjunction with use of cilostazol (a phosphodiesterase III inhibitor), which is licensed for non-critical peripheral arterial disease.

Some areas of arterial disease can be revascularised with percutaneous transluminal angioplasty (PTA). This has the benefits of being minimally invasive and repeatable. Unfortunately long-term results are inferior to bypass surgery and re-stenosis may occur, particularly in smokers, and close follow-up is required. Atherosclerotic occlusion of 10 cm is considered too long for PTA.

For critical and debilitating ischaemia, bypass graft surgery is performed using vein or synthetic (usually ePTFE) graft. Most commonly the long saphenous vein is harvested, or if this not available or of good quality (ie narrow or varicosed) then the short saphenous or, failing that, arm veins can be employed. In bypass surgery ending above the level of the knee, ePTFE and vein have equivalent survival (Table 3.2). However, in low-flow, small (< 6 mm) vessels, synthetic grafts perform poorly and vein is the only option for long-term survival. A vein patch or cuff at the distal anastomosis improves haemodynamics and has been shown to improve patency. Early (< 30 days) graft failure occurs due to thrombosis within the graft, either due to poor suture technique or inadequate distal 'run-off'. The majority of graft failures occur after 12 months due to neointimal hyperplasia, usually most pronounced at the distal anastomosis. Many centres perform graft surveillance programmes to intervene early. Prostacyclin infusion is used in some patients with 'high-risk' anastomoses to try to maintain patency in the early postoperative period.

Table 3.2 Three-year patency of above- and below-knee bypass

	Above knee	**Below knee**
Vein	80–90%	50–70%
ePTFE	70–80%	< 10%

Non-surgical treatments of critical limb ischaemia include: pressure care of extremities, chemical lumbar sympathectomy, dorsal column stimulation and slow-release opioid analgesia. Prostacyclin analogues may have a role in patients with vasospastic disorders.

GANGRENE

Gangrene is tissue necrosis with putrefaction. It may occur following infarction following vascular occlusion, frostbite or trench foot (cold immersion), infection or irradiation.

Examination

- **Dry gangrene** – occurs when necrosed tissue mummifies following infarction. The tissue is black (haemoglobin breakdown) and dry. There is virtually no spread of cellulitis. A zone of demarcation is seen between gangrenous and healthy tissue
- **Gas (wet) gangrene** – implies superadded infection with the spore- and gas-forming anaerobe *Clostridium perfringens*. Pain is severe and the patient is usually septic and unwell. Gas collection in subcutaneous tissue results in crepitus. Cellulitis is seen to spread and no clear demarcation is seen between gangrenous and healthy tissue

Treatment

- Analgesia as required
- **Dry gangrene –** may not need any treatment and the putrefied section will eventually drop off leaving healthy tissue
- **Wet gangrene** – give oxygen and fluid to resuscitate the patient. Broad-spectrum antibiotics including anaerobe cover. Amputation may be required to limit spreading of gangrene
- In both forms, arterial reconstruction may be required to stop progression of gangrene

Acute limb ischaemia occurs due to embolisation, acute thrombosis of an atherosclerotic plaque or thrombosis within a bypass graft (Table 3.3). Unless there has been preceding chronic limb ischaemia with collateral vessel development, there will be insufficient distal blood flow to maintain tissue viability.

Table 3.3 Causes of acute limb ischaemia

Thrombosis	Atherosclerosis Peripheral aneurysm Graft occlusion
Embolism	Atrial fibrillation Ventricular thrombus Valvular vegetation Aneurysm
Other	Popliteal entrapment Extrinsic compression Arterial dissection

The cardinal features of acute arterial occlusion are remembered as the **6 Ps**:

- Pallor
- Paraesthesia
- Paralysis
- Pain
- Pulseless
- Perishing with cold

History

- Duration of symptoms – note that revascularisation of an acutely ischaemic limb that has been hypoxic for some time will result in the introduction of numerous inflammatory mediators into the systemic circulation (ischaemia-reperfusion syndrome). This is a significant cause of morbidity and mortality after restoration of blood flow
- Previous bypass surgery on affected limb – think of graft occlusion

- Risk factors for atherosclerosis and important co-morbidities:

  - Smoking
  - Diabetes
  - Hypertension
  - Hypercholesterolaemia
  - Cardiac disease and symptoms
  - Respiratory disease and symptoms
  - Cerebrovascular disease (strokes or TIA)
  - Previous history of peripheral vascular disease/intervention

- Previous history of intermittent claudication → thrombosis
- Risk factors for embolic occlusion:

  - Known cardiac disease, eg atrial fibrillation or previous myocardial infarction
  - Known aortic or peripheral aneurysm

- Risk factors for spontaneous thrombosis:

  - Use of oral contraception
  - History of previous thrombosis
  - Known history of thrombophilic disorders (eg protein C or S deficiency)

- Home circumstance, mobility and quality of life

Examination

Up to 6 hours of ischaemia will produce a painful, pale limb which may have sensory deficit. After 6 hours, the limb develops mottling and after 12 hours will no longer blanche and will show signs of compartment syndrome.

- General system examination – particularly note cardiac and respiratory systems as these affect perioperative management if surgery is required
- A full vascular examination is important as atherosclerotic and aneurysm disease is often multifocal:

  - Inspection – colour change in limbs; ulceration; scars; mottling
  - Palpate all upper and lower limb pulses. Feel for any thrills overlying large vessels

- ○ Remember that the femoral artery is under the mid-inguinal point (half way between the anterior superior iliac spine (ASIS) and pubic symphysis) and not the mid-point of the inguinal ligament (half way between the ASIS and pubic tubercle – this is the position of the deep inguinal ring)
- ○ Feel for temperature change between both limbs
- ○ Sensation to light touch
- ○ Muscle tenderness and weakness – suggests tissue loss
- ○ Capillary refill at hallux
- ○ Buerger's angle and test

- Hand-held Doppler over peripheral pulses. An absent signal indicates occlusion

Investigations

- U&E, FBC, clotting if on anticoagulants
- Group and save in case theatre is required; crossmatch 4 units blood if decision to operate is made
- CXR – patients are often smokers and have co-existent cardiac and respiratory disease
- ECG
- Arterial USS/duplex or angiography may be available in some centres and at short notice in some centres

Treatment

Acute limb ischaemia and graft occlusion is an emergency. Generally, tissue injury caused by up to 6 hours of ischaemia is generally reversible, whereas after 12 hours it is non-recoverable. A senior opinion must be sought if the clinical suspicion arises, as unnecessary delays may make the situation non-recoverable. In the meantime:

- Analgesia
- Oxygen mask to maximise peripheral perfusion; monitor saturation
- Intravenous access and rehydration
- Urinary catheter and monitor hourly output; maintain output at > 0.5 ml/kg per hour
- Chase blood results and correct abnormalities
- Anticoagulate with heparin:

  - ○ 5000 IU bolus followed by 1250 IU/h iv infusion

> If a patient has had a previous bypass graft and you think it may be
> occluded, it probably is

Embolic disease can be treated immediately by embolectomy with a
Fogarty catheter or intra-arterial infusion of a thrombolytic via a
catheter placed at the clot.

Note that thrombolysis may be complicated by haemorrhage (eg
gastrointestinal, stroke, intra-ocular).

Embolectomy is inadvisable for thrombosis as the intimal trauma will
create further thrombosis, compounding the presenting problem.
Thrombosis of a ruptured atherosclerotic plaque requires intra-arterial
thrombolysis or bypass surgery.

If there is doubt over the aetiology of the cause of the acute ischaemia,
or if an acute plaque/graft thrombosis is suspected then an angiogram
is required. If time is limited, an 'on-table' angiogram is performed by
the surgeon in theatre using a mobile image intensifier. This defines the
anatomy the arterial tree, identifies the aetiology and allows instigation of
thrombolysis or planning of surgery. Sometimes a fasciotomy is required
when there has been prolonged ischaemia to avoid compartment
syndrome (see pages 131–133). Generally, if acute arterial occlusion is
left for longer than 8 hours then irreversible tissue loss ensues.

If there is evidence of irreversible ischaemia then amputation must be
considered as revascularisation will not save the leg but may create
multiorgan failure from ischaemia-reperfusion injury.

CONTRAINDICATIONS FOR THROMBOLYSIS

- Active internal bleeding
- Pregnancy
- Cerebrovascular accident/TIA within 2 months
- Surgery within 2 weeks (craniotomy within 2 months)
- Trauma within 10 days
- Intracerebral tumour
- Known gastrointestinal bleeding tendency

> **SIGNS OF IRREVERSIBLE TISSUE LOSS**
>
> - Calf tenderness
> - Weakness
> - Fixed mottling
> - Sensory loss

THE DIABETIC FOOT

The combination of diabetic neuropathy, large- and small-vessel disease and diabetes-associated co-morbidities (eg hypertension, immune depression) add to make the lower limb extremity at high risk of ulceration, infection, deformity and gangrene.

Particular risk factors for diabetic foot ulceration are:

- Poor blood sugar control
- Age
- Peripheral arterial disease
- Previous ulceration
- Neuropathy
- Altered foot shape
- Social debilitation

In addition, smoking in such individuals considerably worsens prognosis.

History

- Symptoms of neuropathic pain – foot/shin burning or shooting pain, worse at night, better with activity
- Symptoms of ischaemic rest pain – foot burning pain, worse with elevation and activity, better with rest and dependency (hanging leg out of bed)
- Intermittent claudication – calf ache on walking fixed distance, relieved by a few minutes of rest
- Determine type of diabetes and efficacy of control; are there any other complications of diabetes (eg visual, renal)
- Full past medical history, systems review and drug history; document social circumstance and functional ability
- History of foot trauma

Examination

- Full cardiac and vascular examination. Check for bruits over carotid, renal and femoral arteries. Check BP
- Neurological examination of lower limbs. Include vibration, pin prick and proprioception. Describe in terms of dermatomes (see page 282)
- Foot deformity
- Ulceration – describe exact position, size, shape and extent of any cellulitis. Look specifically at pressure areas. Many centres use photographs for documentation
- Ischaemic ulcers are typically sited at the toes, heel and first metatarsal head. Neuropathic ulcerations are punched-out and found in pressure areas
- **Charcot's neurarthropathy** – is characterised by bone and joint destruction with abnormal remodelling. The foot is usually warm and swollen (inflammatory arthropathy). The mid-foot is most affected and there is often collapse of that area producing a 'rocker bottom' foot which is a common site for ulceration

Investigations

- U&E, WCC, HbA1c
- Monitor BM
- X-ray of foot if there is deformity
- Arterial USS and Doppler will give falsely raised ABPI due to arterial calcification. The waveform is often monophasic. Use hallux pressures if there is any doubt
- Arterial duplex and angiography to determine any correctable arterial disease (remember risk of renal function deterioration from contrast medium and interaction with metformin)

Treatment

- Strict glucose monitoring – liaise with diabetologist
- Pressure-relieving dressing and nail care – liaise with podiatrist
- May require angioplasty or bypass surgery as indicated by angiography and patient risk. Non-revascularisable, infected or gangrenous extremity may require amputation

The decision to amputate a limb is not one to be taken lightly. Half of those undergoing amputation for critical limb ischaemia will be dead within a year. Limb amputation is indicated if a limb is 'dead, dying or useless':

- Critical limb ischaemia not amenable to revascularisation
- Massive trauma
- Infection – gas gangrene
- Soft tissue malignancy
- Paralysed limb, eg following polio

When deciding the level for amputation (Table 3.7), a number of factors must be taken into account:

- Perfusion must be adequate to allow healing. If there is poor bleeding at the level of an amputation then it is likely to break down, with resulting morbidity and mortality. Preoperatively, the most appropriate level may be determined clinically and from angiographic data
- Tissue, especially muscle, must be healthy
- Flexure contractures of any joint must be recognised. This is a major disadvantage when trying prosthetic limbs
- The stump must allow fitting of a prosthetic limb without being too tight or loose
- The patient's co-morbidity and baseline mobility state will also influence level of amputation

Table 3.4 Types of amputation

Hind quarter	Involves disarticulation of hip. This is rare and usually used following trauma or for malignancy. Uncommonly it is used for very proximal arterial occlusion
Above knee (trans-femoral)	In critical ischaemia, indicated when the calf is not perfused or when excessive knee joint contracture excludes a trans-tibial amputation. Femur to be left should be around 25 cm. Useful for severe lower limb trauma and proximal vascular disease. Anterior and posterior myofascial lengths are of equal length. Common
Through knee (Gritti–Stokes)	Uncommon, although may be considered when there has already been a contralateral above-knee amputation as the difference in stump lengths allows the patient 'leverage' to move in bed. Disadvantaged by difficulty in fitting prosthesis
Below-knee (trans-tibial)	In critical ischaemia, indicated when calf is perfused, there is no knee joint contracture and mobilisation with a prosthesis is predicated. Tibial stump 10–15 cm with fibula shorter. Long posterior (Burgess) myofascial flap folded forward over tibia end to meet short anterior flap. Common
Ankle Foot – 'ray' amputation	'Syme's amputation' through ankle. Uncommon. Wedge excision of ischaemic tissue to metatarsal level, with the wound packed and left open. This is performed on diabetic patients who have a combination of large and small vessel disease and neuropathy
Trans-metatarsal	For gangrenous toes but well-perfused forefoot

It is important to give antibiotics perioperatively to avoid cellulitis and
C. perfringens infection.

> **COMPLICATIONS**
>
> - Bleeding
> - Infection/gas gangrene/osteomyelitis
> - Ischaemia
> - Wound dehiscence
> - Pain/neuroma – important to cut nerves proximally
> - Phantom limb
> - Psychological

Any postoperative amputee with evidence of shock (tachycardia, hypotension or reduced urine output) needs senior review. Note whether an epidural is being used as this may also be a cause of hypotension. Check dressing for blood 'strike through' and make a note of drain output if one is present. While you are waiting for senior review, institute resuscitation measures: oxygen, good iv access, colloid or normal saline infusion (avoid 5% dextrose as this will redistribute into all fluid compartments). Make sure that there is a urinary catheter. Check Hb, U&E, ECG and ensure that a group and save/crossmatch sample has been sent.

Phantom limb pain occurs in 50–80% of cases. Treatment includes pregabalin, gabapentin, carbamazepine or transcutaneous nerve stimulation. Liaison with a pain specialist is valuable. Tight, elasticated bandages should not be used In vascular amputees due to the risk of ischaemia.

COMPARTMENT SYNDROME

This is **a limb-threatening emergency**. Compartment syndrome occurs when perfusion pressure falls below tissue pressure in a closed anatomical space. Reperfusion of a limb following prolonged ischaemia results in profound limb swelling. Since the limbs are composed of muscle enclosed within non-compliant osteo-fascial compartments (in the leg these are: lateral, anterior, posterior and deep posterior), an elevation in pressure cannot be accommodated and results in compression of vascular and neuronal structures.

Compartment syndrome occurs when intra-compartment pressure exceeds 30 mmHg. As the pressure rises, venous flow and nerve function first deteriorate followed by reduced arterial inflow. Muscle death is inevitable after 6 hours unless the facial compartment is opened and allowed to decompress. This operation is known as a fasciotomy – longitudinal incisions through skin and fascia allow pressure within all compartments to be released.

If treatment is delayed, the leg may become irretrievable, leading to amputation, hyperkalaemia and myoglobinaemia.

History

- History of injury – mechanism and injury sustained

  ○ High energy, crush
  ○ Fractures

- Recent revascularisation
- Ask about the 6 Ps of acute ischaemia (see page 123)

  ○ Pain and paraesthesia are classic features
  ○ Other Ps are late symptoms/signs
  ○ Pain is out of proportion to injury and often resistant to analgesia and worse with movement

- Anticoagulation – increases risk of compartment syndrome

Examination

- Pain heightened by passive movement of muscles in the compartment
- Tender or indurated muscle compartment
- Distal sensory disturbance
- Scars from injury or surgery
- Erythema – venous congestion
- Reduced capillary re-fill
- Absent pulses occurs after muscle compartment has necrosed

Investigations

- Measurement of compartment pressures

  ○ Venflon or spinal needle
  ○ Attach to pressure monitor used for arterial pressure monitoring
  ○ Measure all compartments

- Check baseline renal function

Treatment

- Oxygen
- Fluid resuscitation and maintain hydration
- Urgent senior review
- Fasciotomy required if pressure is > 30 mmHg or the difference between the diastolic and compartment pressure is < 30mmHg

---

CAUSES OF COMPARTMENT SYNDROME

Increase fluid in compartment

- Reperfusion injury
- Trauma (fracture, haemorrhage)
- Intensive muscle use (eg tetany, vigorous exercise, seizures)
- Burns
- Envenomation
- Decreased serum osmolarity (eg nephrotic syndrome)
- Infiltrated infusion

Decreased compartment size

- Military anti-shock trousers (MAST)
- Casts

ANEURYSMS

Aneurysms are defined as abnormal dilatation of an artery – by greater than 50% its normal diameter. Progressive dilatation of the aneurysm sac eventually results in rupture and haemorrhage.

Aneurysms are described as either true or false. A true aneurysm is a dilation of the whole thickness of the vessel wall. The most common cause is degeneration of the vessel wall by atherosclerosis. These are most common in men and have risk factors common to all cardiovascular diseases (smoking, hypertension, diabetes mellitus, hypercholesterolaemia, family history, homocystinaemia). True aneurysms may also be congenital (eg Berry aneurysms) or associated with connective tissue diseases (eg Ehlers–Danlos, Marfan's), infections (salmonella, tuberculosis) and inflammatory disorders (Takayasu's disease). These patients have co-morbidities and attention has to be given to past medical history, current medication and systems review.

A false aneurysm occurs when the vessel wall is injured and blood becomes contained by thrombus and surrounding tissues, with eventual formation of a sac communicating with the artery. The wall of the aneurysm may consist of haematoma, making it prone to rupture, eg common femoral artery false aneurysm following repeated injections by drug misusers.

COMPLICATIONS OF ANEURYSMAL DISEASE

- Rupture
- Embolism
- Ischaemia
- Thrombosis
- Dissection
- Pressure effects

ABDOMINAL AORTIC ANEURYSM

Ninety-five per cent of AAAs occur below the level of the renal arteries. Most consider an aortic diameter > 3 cm to be aneurysmal. AAAs cause 1.3% of deaths in men > 65 years. Overall mortality following rupture is 65–85% with approximately 50% of AAA ruptures resulting in immediate death. Conversely, elective surgery has a mortality of < 5%, and thus it is a prophylactic treatment for rupture. Rate of growth is initially slow but exponentially increases with increasing aneurysm diameter. Remember that management of co-morbidity is of equal importance as the aneurysm, as most patients do not die of AAA rupture but of co-existing pathology.

In approximately 10% of cases there is a dense inflammatory reaction surrounding the aneurysm sac. Such 'inflammatory aneurysms' are not managed differently but can produce more symptoms and are more challenging to operate.

Always be cautious when a > 60-year-old man is referred with 'renal colic' – this should be considered to be an AAA unless proved otherwise.

Table 3.5 Risk of rupture of AAA in 1 year

< 4 cm	0%
4–5 cm	0–5%
5–6 cm	3–15%
6–7 cm	10–20%
7–8 cm	20–40%
> 8 cm	30–50%

History

- Majority of unruptured AAA are asymptomatic
- Occasionally AAA may present with acute lower limb ischaemia following embolisation of thrombus or aortic occlusion
- Back pain in isolation or upper/central abdominal pain which radiates to back – this suggests sac expansion and is an indication for urgent repair (see later)
- Malaise and weight loss suggest an inflammatory aneurysm
- Find out how the aneurysm was diagnosed – find out size and extent (infrarenal or suprarenal)
- Ask for risk factors:

  ○ Smoker – AAA is four times more common in smokers
  ○ Hypertension
  ○ Hypercholesterolaemia
  ○ Diabetes mellitus
  ○ Family history of cardiovascular diseases

- Pay close attention to past medical, surgical and drug history
- Any symptoms suggestive of intermittent claudication, TIA/cerebrovascular accident
- Review of systems – pay particular attention to cardiac and respiratory symptoms (exertional chest pain, palpitations, dyspnoea, orthopnoea)
- Social history – baseline functional ability

Examination

- Full systems examination – focus on respiratory and cardiac
- Check all peripheral and central pulses, and listen for overlying bruits. Pay particular attention to lower limb pulses and document your findings clearly. This is important, as one risk of AAA surgery is distal embolisation of thrombus

- Bimanual examination of supraumbilical area – remember that the aortic bifurcation is at L4, just below the umbilicus. Check for expansibility and pulsatility
- 69% of AAA that are 4.0–4.9 cm and 90% of AAA > 5.0 cm are palpable
- There is often co-existence with aneurysms of the popliteal (40%) and common femoral (25%) arteries

Investigations

Diagnosis

- AXR – can show calcification within aortic wall. This is usually an incidental finding and AXR is a poor diagnostic tool
- USS – accurate, simple, cheap. Used as a first-line investigation in the elective setting and for screening
- CT – used to determine whether endovascular (see below) treatment is possible. Provides anatomical information including: angulation, size of AAA neck, and amount of thrombus within sac. It will also visualise whether it is inflammatory or not. In the emergent setting, provided that the patient is haemodynamically stable enough, CT is employed to confirm leak/rupture. The 'crescent sign' – blood flow within sac thrombus – is a sign of imminent rupture
- Angiogram – less commonly used. Still used in some centres as part of work up for endovascular stenting. Will give information of iliac arteries (important consideration for stent delivery)
- MR angiogram – uncommonly used

Admitted for elective repair

- U&E – renal dysfunction related to diabetes, hypertension, renal artery involvement. Uretero-hydronephrosis can occur with inflammatory AAA
- FBC, crossmatch as per departmental guidelines, clotting
- Raised ESR suggests an inflammatory aneurysm – although this is not routinely checked in most departments
- CXR, ECG, blood sugar, cholesterol
- Full cardiology assessment is needed if there is a cardiac history or symptoms. This may include echocardiogram or thallium scan. Some patients will need coronary artery angiography/stenting. Remember that 40–60% will have co-existing cardiac disease

Note: Make sure that any CT scans are available to go down to theatre with patient and liaise with anaesthetist in advance to organise a postoperative ITU/HDU bed.

Treatment

Curative treatment is surgery but medical risk reduction cannot be overlooked.

Medical

- Reduction of risk factors, eg stop smoking, control of hypertension
- Antiplatelet medication
- Statins

Surgical

The decision to operate is determined by the risk of rupture, presence of complications and patient's fitness for surgery. Most patients do not die of their aneurysm, so the decision to operate is individualised to the patient.

INDICATIONS FOR AAA REPAIR

- Rupture/contained retroperitoneal haematoma – immediate repair
- Tender/abdominal/back pain – suggests impending rupture – urgent repair
- Asymptomatic > 5.5 cm
- Embolisation
- Thrombosis
- Ureteric obstruction
- >1 cm/year rate of growth

Those with AAA under 5 cm undergo 6-monthly USS screening as an outpatient (3-monthly in some centres if > 4.5 cm). Work-up for surgery is started when > 5.0 cm and performed when > 5.5 cm.

Open surgery/conventional repair

This is done through a midline, transverse or retroperitoneal approach. A small number of centres are now performing laparoscopic aortic surgery. The aneurysm sac is opened and a Dacron tube or bifurcated graft placed in an inlay manner. The sac is sutured back over the graft to provide coverage. The advantage of the open method is that it provides a cure with no need for long-term follow-up, unlike endovascular stent (see below). It is, however, major surgery with a mortality up to 5%.

COMPLICATIONS OF AORTIC SURGERY

- Haemorrhage
- Spinal ischaemia
- Stroke
- Colonic ischaemia
- Myocardial infarction
- DIC
- Renal failure

- ARDS
- Graft thrombosis
- False aneurysm
- Graft infection
- Aorto-enteric fistula
- Distal embolism
- Erectile dysfunction

Endovascular aneurysm repair

Endovascular aneurysm repair (EVAR) was first introduced in 1991 and involves placement of a covered stent endoluminally, via the common femoral artery, under fluoroscopic guidance. Only approximately 60% of AAA will be anatomically suitable for EVAR. Proponents claim that avoidance of aortic clamping, large incision and colonic ischaemia during EVAR reduce morbidity and mortality. The major disadvantage of EVAR is that the aneurysm may still grow and rupture if the stent-graft migrates, if there is back flow of blood into the sac or mechanical failure of the graft (these are termed 'endoleaks'). Unlike open surgery, close long-term follow-up with serial CT or USS is required to detect endoleaks.

RUPTURED AAA

If this is suspected, inform your senior straight away. The main differential diagnoses are acute pancreatitis, intestinal ischaemia and gastrointestinal perforation. Refer to section on the assessment of abdominal pain (pages 35–40).

History

- Sudden-onset abdominal pain radiating to back. Back pain may be the dominant feature. Pain may radiate to flanks and scrotum
- Collapse

- Is there a know history of AAA – under follow-up?
- Risk factors for vascular disease, past medical history and social history as above

Examination

- ABC ATLS assessment and simultaneous resuscitation
- Shock – ↑ respiratory rate, ↑ pulse, ↓ BP
- Cold periphery, pale, anxious
- ↓ Urine output
- Abdominal tenderness, bloating
- Flank bruising
- Pulsatile/expansile mass – tender
- Lower limb pulses – may be absent

Investigations

- U&E, FBC, clotting
- Amylase
- Crossmatch 6 units blood if there is a strong suspicion
- ECG
- If stable enough – CXR and CT scan (the gold standard – preferable to USS)

A patient should not be transferred to CT scanner if not stabilised – they will arrest in the scan department otherwise. Similarly, if there is a high index of suspicion, surgery should not be delayed for radiological investigations.

Treatment

- Oxygen
- Large iv cannula – no smaller than green (18 gauge) and ideally grey (16 gauge); normal saline and colloid (not 5% dextrose) fast infusion
- Get blood ASAP and start blood transfusion
- Analgesia
- Urinary catheter
- **Theatre immediately**. Open repair remains the standard. A few centres are now doing emergency EVAR but the role of this is under evaluation

POPLITEAL ANEURYSM

This is the second most common aneurysm and most common peripheral aneurysm. Most people consider a 2-cm popliteal artery to be an aneurysm. It may cause chronic ischaemia due to thrombosis, acute ischaemia from embolisation, pain by compressing adjacent structures and rupture. Half are bilateral, and in 40% cases there is an associated AAA.

History

- Most are asymptomatic and are found incidentally
- 40% are associated with AAA – see above
- Ask about both legs
- Claudication – distance, is this stable or deteriorating?
- Symptoms of acute ischaemia – the 6 Ps (see page 123)
- Past medical history as above
- Social history – degree of independence may affect management

Examination

- Full system examination. Check all peripheral and central pulses. In particular look for co-existing AAAs and contralateral aneurysms
- The popliteal pulse is usually difficult to feel unless patient is very skinny. If you can feel a popliteal pulse – particularly in a large leg – then the patient probably has an aneurysm!
- Check for evidence of critical ischaemia of a distal extremity

Investigations

- General medical investigation as for aortic aneurysm above
- Duplex USS of popliteal artery
- Angiogram – will demonstrate distal run-off

Treatment

Surgery is carried out for symptomatic aneurysms. Small aneurysms < 2.5 cm are screened every 3–6 months. Aneurysms of 2.5–3.0 cm or greater should be repaired electively. The timing of intervention depends on acuteness of presentation. An acutely ischaemic limb will need urgent intervention. Treatment options are:

- Exclusion and bypass: the aneurysm is ligated on both sides and a bypass performed using a vein graft. This is the most common treatment. Distal run off vessel is required

- Thrombolysis – is performed for acutely thrombosed artery to re-establish flow
- Amputation – is performed if the aneurysm becomes occluded and there is no distal vessel flow for successful bypass

CEREBROVASCULAR DISEASE

Stroke is the third commonest cause of death after coronary artery disease and malignancy. Of all cerebral ischaemic infarcts, 20–30% are due to atheroma of the major extracranial and intracranial cerebral blood vessels, most commonly due to atherosclerosis of the internal carotid artery at the level of the carotid bifurcation. 30% of strokes are cardiac in origin, but cardiac causes predominate in younger patients.

Atherosclerotic plaque destabilisation results in embolisation of debris from its central core, resulting in symptoms. The risk of developing symptoms increases with the severity of carotid stenosis. Thus, the basis for carotid endarterectomy is to remove a stenosing plaque from the internal carotid artery origin to alleviate the risk of cerebral embolisation. A completely occluded artery is a stable situation, since absence of blood flow obviates any risk of distal embolisation.

History

Symptomatic carotid stenoses will manifest in one of three ways:

- **Stroke**: acute focal loss of neurological function with symptoms exceeding > 24 hours, or resulting in death, with no cause other than of vascular origin. Classic carotid territory manifestations include hemi-motor and hemi-sensory signs, monocular visual loss and higher cortical dysfunction (eg dysphagia)
- **Transient ischaemic attack**: acute focal loss of neurological function with symptoms lasting < 24 hours with no persistent deficit. The risk of stroke following TIA is up to 17% within 1 year. TIAs commonly occur in clusters due to the appearance of friable thrombus at the carotid bifurcation
- **Amaurosis fugax**: transient painless, monocular loss of vision, which may be total or sectorial. It is classically described as a 'curtain falling across the eye'

A left-sided stroke or TIA may result in aphasia or language disturbance, although right cerebral hemisphere speech dominance is seen in left-handed individuals.

Cerebrovascular events have risk factors common with all atherosclerotic processes: hypertension, smoking, diabetes mellitus, hypercholesterolaemia, male sex and increasing age.

There are additionally frequent co-morbidities. Enquire about ischaemic heart disease, peripheral vascular disease, COPD and renal disease. There may be a history of previous strokes or TIAs.

Enquire for the presence of any alternative sources of embolism such as atrial fibrillation, heart valve disease or myocardial infarction. Check drug history for anticoagulation or clopidogrel use that will have to be stopped prior to surgery.

Examination

- A full neurological examination is required to provide baseline information prior to undergoing surgery. This is particularly important given the small risk of intraoperative stroke
- **Carotid bruit** is an inaccurate sign; 12% of the general population over 60 years will have an audible bruit, although 50–75% of patients with symptomatic carotid stenoses will not

Investigations

Once TIA, stroke or amaurosis fugax is diagnosed, precipitous patient work-up is required as a major cerebrovascular event may be impending.

- Carotid duplex ultrasound: determines degree of carotid stenosis or occlusion in both arteries and provides anatomical information
- Intra-arterial contrast or magnetic resonance angiography: indicated to confirm carotid occlusion and if there is suspicion of atherosclerosis in the proximal vessel near the aortic arch

Given the likelihood of cardiac and respiratory co-morbidity, a full work-up is required as described in Chapter 1. This should include ECG, CXR, U&E and FBC (to exclude polycythaemia and anaemia), glucose, lipids and sickle cell screen. Echocardiography and pulmonary function tests should also be considered. Liaise with the anaesthetist if a preoperative patient has significant risk factors for surgery.

Treatment

Medical

- Risk-factor management by smoking cessation, treatment of hypertension and strict diabetes control
- Aspirin for asymptomatic and symptomatic stenosis
- Aspirin is often combined with dipyridamole in symptomatic disease
- Clopidogrel used if intolerant or co-existing cardiac disease
- Statins
- Angina and atrial fibrillation treatment should be optimised by co-operation with a cardiologist

Carotid endarterectomy

Carotid endarterectomy (CEA) is the standard surgical treatment for symptomatic, significant carotid disease. CEA entails exposure of the carotid bifurcation and internal carotid origin via an incision along the medial border of the sternocleidomastoid. Following arteriotomy at the carotid bifurcation and careful removal of the atherosclerotic plaque (endarterectomy), the carotid artery is closed with a patch to prevent narrowing. Recent evidence has suggested that CEA may be of benefit for asymptomatic, significant carotid stenoses in selected cases.

Table 3.6 Complications of CEA

Wound	Infection Bruising Great auricular nerve injury (makes shaving difficult)
Cranial nerve injury	Hypoglossal Glossopharyngeal Less commonly – mandibular branch of facial nerve, vagus, spinal part of accessory nerve
Perioperative stroke	Up to 4%

continued

Table 3.6 *Continued*

Bleeding	Uncommon but always be wary of the possibility. **Significant bleeding may cause tracheal compression, stridor and respiratory arrest**. Rapidly expanding haematoma needs urgent senior attention, opening of the skin and platysma, and exploration in theatre. Call the crash team if there is evidence of airway compromise
Recurrent stenosis	1.5–4.5%

Stenting

Carotid stenting is a less invasive procedure than CEA. This is carried out percutaneously under local anaesthetic and involves passing a balloon catheter over a guide wire to pre-dilate the narrowed carotid artery before insertion of a metal stent, which maintains patency. A cerebral protection device may also be used in this procedure to prevent particles dislodged during the stenting procedure from passing into the cerebral circulation. However, uncertainty remains over its long-term success, wider applicability and the perceived risk of iatrogenic stroke, which will be addressed in forthcoming studies.

VENOUS DISEASE

DEEP VEIN THROMBOSIS

Ninety-five per cent of DVTs originate in the lower limbs around valve sinuses in the calf. DVT and subsequent pulmonary embolism is a major cause of postoperative morbidity and mortality. Furthermore, a fifth of DVTs will result in a post-thrombotic limb. Unless contraindicated, all patients require DVT prophylaxis. If there is any suspicion of a DVT, then this must be investigated and treated promptly.

The pathogenesis of DVTs is described by **Virchow's triad**:

- Venous stasis
- Hypercoagulability
- Vessel wall damage

This triad predicts all predisposing factors to DVTs (Table 3.6).

Table 3.7 Risk factors for DVT

Venous stasis	Immobility, eg long haul flight, paralysis Recent surgery Pelvis mass Pregnancy Obesity
Hypercoagulability	Malignancy Myeloproliferative disease Oral contraceptive pill Factor V Leiden mutation Protein C deficiency Protein S deficiency Antithrombin III deficiency Homocystinuria Nephrotic syndrome Smoking
Vessel wall damage	Previous DVT Trauma/surgery Indwelling catheters (eg central lines)

DVT below the level of the knee has a low risk of embolisation, unlike above-knee variants. Most DVTs are asymptomatic. The most common presenting features are isolated leg swelling, calf discomfort, erythema and dilated superficial veins. On occasion the first presentation will be following a pulmonary embolism (pleuritic chest pain, dyspnoea, collapse).

PROXIMAL DVT (ILIO-FEMORAL SEGMENT)

History

Symptoms

- Swelling of limb – unilateral as concomitant bilateral DVT, although possible, is uncommon
- Muscle tenderness – unilateral
- Increase pain with movement of limb
- Pain worse when limb dependent, eased when elevated
- Pleuritic chest pain, dyspnoea, palpitations → suggests embolisation

Predisposition

- Previous DVT/PE
- Contraceptive pill, HRT use
- Smoking
- Previous/recent surgery
- Current or previous malignancy
- Known coagulation disorder
- Previous limb injury
- Recent long-distance travel/immobility

Examination

- Warm, unilateral swelling – pitting oedema
- Erythema
- Measure limb diameter 10 cm below tibial tuberosity with tape and compare with the other side
- Muscle tenderness in compression. Ilio-femoral DVT may cause groin tenderness
- Calf pain on passive dorsiflexion (Homan's sign) is inadvisable due to risk of embolisation; accuracy of this test is 50%
- Limb or abdominal scars to suggest recent or previous surgery
- Abdominal and pelvic examination (including rectal examination) to exclude pelvic pathology

Phlegmasia alba dolens = white painful leg. This is due to iliofemoral thrombosis.

Phlegmasia cerulea dolens = purple painful leg. Distal extension of a proximal DVT to occlude small collateral veins leading to swelling, engorgement and limitation of arterial inflow due to back pressure. This is extremely painful and limb loss is a high risk.

Investigations

- D-dimer (fibrinogen degradation product) – if positive then USS is required; USS still advisable if negative but there is a high clinical suspicion
- USS including venous duplex
- Venography – now uncommon
- If appropriate look for predisposing cause:
  - Clotting screen
  - Investigate for malignancy – especially pelvic
  - Pro-coagulant screen (discuss with haematologist)

Treatment

- TEDS – avoid if there is severe arterial insufficiency
- LMWH
- Intraoperative calf compression stocking
- Early mobilisation
- Ensure hydration
- Discontinue OCP
- Clinical suspicion of DVT warrants empirical treatment with LMWH, with dose based on patient weight, while investigations are awaited
- Below-knee DVT may be treated with low-dose prophylactic LMWH dose with TEDS until patient is mobile. Some clinicians prefer full anticoagulation even though risk of embolisation is relatively low
- Above-knee DVT requires full anticoagulation with warfarin and temporary LMWH until INR is in therapeutic range; maintain warfarin INR at 2–3
- Recurrent DVT may require long-term anticoagulation
- Proximal/pelvic DVT or recurrent DVTs may require placement of an inferior vena cave filter to prevent pulmonary embolism
- Thrombolysis for occlusive DVT causing venous gangrene in extremity

POST-PHLEBITIC SYNDROME

Following re-cannulisation of a thrombosed deep vein there may be destruction of valve leading to valvular incompetence and distal venous hypertension. This results in thickening of the vein, impedance to arterial inflow, and extravasation of erythrocytes and leukocytes into surrounding tissue. This then results in a local inflammatory response, oedema and fibrosis. Eventually skin may breakdown, particularly in the 'gaiter' area around the medial malleolus, leading to pigmentation, eczema and venous ulceration. Ulceration usually starts 2–3 years after venous injury.

History

- History of DVT/symptoms of DVT
- Previous pelvic surgery of limb fracture
- History of venous surgery
- How long ulcer has been present
- History of peripheral arterial disease or symptoms consistent with claudication – this is important as the use of compression dressing may make peripheral disease worse

Examination

- Oedema
- Venous eczema
- Pigmentation
- Ulceration – gaiter area
- Pain worse with limb dependent
- Lipodermatosclerosis of pretibial regions

Investigations

- Arterial and deep vein ultrasound plus duplex to assess deep vein competence and make sure that the patient will tolerate compression stocking without compromise to the arterial inflow
- ABPI (Table 3.1) for compression stockings should be > 0.8

Treatment

- Clean ulceration
- Excise necrotic tissue
- Graduated compression stockings, eg 2-, 3- or 4-layer bandage
- Compression stockings should not be used if ABPI is < 0.8

VARICOSE VEINS

These are tortuous, dilated, elongated veins which are associated with valvular incompetence. Varicose veins affect 20–45% of the population. Most are asymptomatic with loss of cosmesis the only complaint.

Varicose veins are classified as primary or secondary. Remember that the superficial (long and short saphenous veins) are connected with the deep venous system by three valved communications:

- Perforator veins
- Sapheno-femoral junction
- Sapheno-popliteal junction

Varicose veins arise when the valves within one or more of these communications becomes incompetent. Surgical treatment of varicose veins is dependent on identifying the site(s) of valve incompetence. Varicose vein surgery is contraindicated where there is a previous history of DVT. If there is doubt, or where there are strong risk factors for DVT, then deep venous incompetence must be excluded. Similarly, where there is a history of previous venous surgery, a venous duplex is required to locate the site of valvular incompetence.

History
- Previous varicose vein surgery
- Previous DVT/symptoms of DVT
- Previous limb fracture/pelvic surgery
- Oral contraception/hormone replacement
- Anticoagulant use
- Symptoms from limb

Examination
- Expose both legs completely. Ask patient to demonstrate veins while standing
- Note areas of varicosities and describe these as either above or below the knee and their distribution
- Note oedema or skin changes suggesting chronic venous hypertension
- Note any scars suggesting previous fracture or varicose vein surgery (the scar will be either at the groin or behind the knee and there may be small avulsion site scars often along the medial aspect of leg)

- Is there a saphena varix? This is a varicosity of the sapheno-femoral junction at the groin. It disappears on lying and is reducible – it is often misdiagnosed as a hernia. It signifies sapheno-femoral junction incompetence and will be associated with varicosities distally in the distribution of the long saphenous vein

Tourniquet test: position the patient supine, elevate the leg and tighten a tourniquet high around the upper thigh. Ask patient to stand. If no varicose veins appear then the site of incompetence is above the tourniquet. If veins appear then move tourniquet down the limb and repeat.

Hand-held Doppler: this is performed more commonly than Trendelenburg's test. Ask the patient to stand. Hold the probe over the sapheno-femoral junction medial to the femoral pulse. Squeeze the calf. If there is a sound of blood going back down the leg on release of the calf then the sapheno-femoral junction is the site of valvular incompetence.

Investigations

In uncomplicated cases, no special investigations are required. A venous ultrasound and duplex is required to identify the site of valve incompetence if there is doubt in the clinical examination or there has been previous varicose vein surgery. If there is any history suggestive of a previous DVT, deep vein USS is required.

Treatment

- Weight loss, smoking cessation
- If asymptomatic it is best to treat non-operatively. Some centres advocate injection sclerotherapy, but risk of recurrence is high
- Support stockings
- Surgery involves disconnection of incompetent valve and stripping of affected vein
- Recent techniques include intraluminal laser ablation and sclerosing foam injection

COMPLICATIONS OF VARICOSE VEINS

- Thrombosis
- Thrombophlebitis
- Itching and aching towards the end of the day
- Bleeding (late)
- Ulceration (late)

CAUSES OF VARICOSE VEINS

Primary

- Due to weakness of vein wall
- Often familial

Secondary

- DVT
- Obstruction to venous outflow (eg pregnancy, pelvic mass)
- High venous pressure, eg arteriovenous fistula

CHAPTER 4

UROLOGY

A CARTER AND R NAPIER HEMY

Symptoms from the lower urinary tract are broadly classified as either **filling** or **voiding** (Table 4.1). Voiding symptoms are most often seen in men with prostatic enlargement. Voiding symptoms are often caused by urinary tract infections, eg cystitis, pyelonephritis.

Other symptoms in urological disorders:

- Loin/back/suprapubic pain
- Incontinence
- Testicular pain
- Haematuria
- Penile discharge
- Suprapubic pain
- Vomiting
- Rigors
- Weight loss

In women it is also worth taking an obstetric history as childbirth can damage the pelvic floor and cause urinary incontinence.

Table 4.1 Classification of urinary tract symptoms

Lower urinary tract symptoms	
Filling (storage)	**Voiding**
Hesitancy (delay in starting to void)	Frequency
Dribbling	Urgency
Intermittency	Nocturia
Pain	Dysuria (stinging/burning)
Poor stream	Strangury (feeling of
Overflow incontinence	incomplete evacuation)
Upper urinary tract symptoms	
Usually pain radiation from loin to groin	
Note: classic colic is different from loin pain associated with infection	

KIDNEY-URETER-BLADDER X-RAY

Essentially, this is a supine plain AXR that includes the kidneys, ureters and bladder (KUB). In addition to providing the same information that a plain AXR would, it is specifically requested to view the renal outline and positions, renal/ureteric calculi, renal calcification and vertebral abnormalities that could affect bladder function. Remember that the kidneys and the bladder soft tissue shadows should be visible on the KUB and that 90% of renal calculi are radio-opaque. The ureters may be traced from the kidney shadow (L1/L2, the left kidney lying higher than the right) down along the tips of the transverse spinous processes, along the sacroiliac joint and then follow roughly the curve of the sacrum to enter into the bladder at the level of the ischial spines (close to the sacroiliac joint). In women of childbearing age, a pregnancy test should be done before taking X-rays.

INTRAVENOUS UROGRAM

Intravenous urogram (IVU) is possibly the easiest-to-interpret means of viewing the anatomy of the urinary tract. It also gives some hint about the function of the kidneys. After an initial, baseline KUB is taken, an intravenous contrast medium is given which is excreted via the kidneys. Repeat KUB films are taken typically after 5 and 20 minutes post-contrast to visualise contrast excretion. Additional delayed films may be taken if there is an obstruction. If there is concern regarding bladder emptying, post-micturition films may also be taken.

As an iv contrast medium is used there is a small risk of contrast allergy and renal function impairment. Metformin should be stopped 2 days before to avoid lactic acidosis. IVU is contraindicated during pregnancy.

ULTRASOUND SCAN

Renal USS can be used to assess kidney size and presence of tumour, cyst, abscess, stones, hydronephrosis and ureteric distension. It is the investigation of choice for patients with renal failure and pyelonephritis. Additional Doppler scanning can detect renal vein thrombosis and arterial flow (important for transplanted kidneys). USS also gives information regarding bladder volume and bladder wall pathology. Sometimes it is difficult to obtain useful images in very obese patients.

Scrotal USS is excellent at visualising testicular/scrotal swellings. Doppler can be used to determine blood flow. This is, however, operator dependent and not always available when needed.

Transrectal ultrasound (TRUS) visualises the prostate and surrounding anatomy. TRUS is used diagnostically to investigate carcinoma of the prostate, often following a raised prostate-specific antigen (PSA). Under these circumstances TRUS-guided biopsies are taken usually after injection of local anaesthetic around the apex of the prostate. Less commonly, TRUS is used to evaluate prostate volume and to investigate azoospermia. It is also used during therapeutic procedures, eg brachytherapy of prostate carcinoma or abscess aspiration. Relative contraindications are painful perianal conditions and active sepsis. TRUS and biopsy are associated with significant morbidity and even potential mortality.

COMPUTED TOMOGRAPHY

Modern CT scanners now can give the best quality information about the urinary tract. They are safe and subject the patient to a radiation dose only just more than that of an average IVU. Non-contrast CT scanning is probably the best option for investigation of suspected ureteric colic. Even radiolucent stones show up on CT scanning and can easily be seen in the ureter to confirm a diagnosis. It can also show possible non-urological causes for the pain such as diverticular disease, biliary colic or a symptomatic/leaking aortic aneurysm. CT scanning should be the first line investigation for urological trauma in a stabilised patient. It is used routinely in the staging of urological malignancies. Interventional radiologists use it to guide biopsy or drainage needles.

MAGNETIC RESONANCE IMAGING

MRI gives better images of the lower urinary tract and pelvic organs than CT and so is preferable in the staging of bladder and prostate cancer. MR urography using gadolinium as a contrast agent is safe for use in the investigation of loin pain in the second trimester of pregnancy. MR is unsafe in the first trimester and physically impossible in the third.

RADIOISOTOPE SCINTIGRAPHY

- ^{99m}Tc-DMSA: Technetium 99m (^{99m}Tc) Dimercaptosuccinic acid (DMSA) binds to functioning renal tubules and so is used as a renal cortical imaging agent. Reduced take-up (photopenia) is seen in areas of scarring (eg after pyelonephritis). It gives the best estimate of differential renal function
- ^{99m}Tc-MAG-3: Mercapto acetyl triglycine (MAG) is filtered and secreted by the kidneys. It is the best agent for evaluating whether there is obstruction to urine flow from the kidney to the bladder. Handling of the radioisotope by both kidneys is plotted against time (a renogram)
- ^{99m}Tc-DPTA: Diethylenetriaminepentaacetic acid (DTPA) can be used in the same way as MAG-3, but does not give quite as good images
- ^{99m}Tc-MDP bone scan: Mercapto diphosphonate (MDP) labelled with a radio-isotope is taken up by any areas of increased bone turnover. In urology it is primarily used to look for the presence of prostate cancer metastases in bone. Prostate cancer tends to cause sclerotic metastases rather than lytic ones. These show up because of the increased bone turnover as hot areas on the bone scan. Other causes of increased bone turnover, such as a healing fracture, osteomyelitis, Paget's disease and bone adjacent to arthritic joints, will also show up

RETROGRADE/MICTURATING CYSTOGRAM

Contrast medium is introduced into the bladder via a urinary catheter. Retrograde cystography in this way is used to detect any leakage of medium from the bladder if there has been any suspected injury. For micturating cystography, the catheter is removed and the bladder screened as the patient is asked to void. This is used to detect vesico-ureteric reflux.

EDTA CLEARANCE

Sequential blood sampling to follow rate of clearance of EDTA from the blood is the best practical means of estimating the glomerular filtration rate (GFR). It is more accurate that creatinine clearance.

Ureteric colic is severe pain associated with the passage of solid, crystalline material, most commonly a calculus (stone) arising from the kidney, along the ureter.

- More common in young adults 20–50 years. Lifetime risk of developing a stone is about 5%
- 90% are idiopathic. Remainder are secondary to hyperparathyroidism, vitamin D excess, primary hyperoxaluria and other metabolic abnormalities
- Half will recur
- Stones < 4 mm in size often pass spontaneously
- Although most calculi are asymptomatic, renal and ureteric stones can be excruciating and can mimic most causes of abdominal pain (see pages 35–40, Abdominal pain, for list of differential diagnoses)
- Complications include:

  - Obstruction and hydronephrosis
  - Renal failure – particularly with staghorn calculi
  - Ureteric stricture
  - Infection (acute infection in an obstructed kidney is a surgical emergency)

Bladder calculi are unusual in the Western world. They are more often found in the 'developing' world secondary to schistosomiasis. They can be seen in the Western world as a response to chronic infection and the presence of foreign bodies such as catheters and sutures. Long-standing bladder stones are a risk factor for the development of squamous cell carcinoma.

Note: Be wary of patients above the age of 50 with ureteric colic! Make sure that this is not a misdiagnosed ruptured AAA. Loin pain is ALWAYS due to a leaking AAA until proved otherwise.

History

- Colicky pain in the loin radiating to the groin/scrotum/labia
- Often associated with vomiting, haematuria, 'filling' and/or 'voiding' urinary symptoms
- Ask about family history of stones, previous history of stones and previous urological instrumentation
- Renal calculi may be asymptomatic
- Pain may settle following passage of the stone

Examination

Patients are often restless with loin tenderness, but comfortable between attacks. They may have a temperature. Perform a thorough abdominal examination to exclude other causes of abdominal pain – classically renal colic is associated with few abdominal signs. It is essential to exclude an AAA in anyone, particularly males, above the age of 50.

Investigations

- Urine dipstick (90% have haematuria) and MSU for culture and sensitivity
- Pregnancy test in women
- Blood tests – WCC, U&E, CRP, glucose, amylase, serum calcium, urate, blood cultures
- 24-hour urinary calcium, oxalate, phosphate, urate, citrate and volume should be reserved for complex stones cases. These are patients with multiple stones, recurring stones or radiolucent stones

- An initial KUB is essential as 90% are radio-opaque and simple KUB can be used for follow up of these patients (see page 150)
- IVU or CT scan, depending on local availability, will be needed to further assess the stone and plan treatment. CT scanning is the most modern way of assessing acute loin pain. It has the advantages of avoiding iv contrast and being able to diagnose non-urological causes of pain

Treatment

Analgesia: Renal colic is **excruciatingly** painful. Non-steroidal analgesia is particularly effective in renal colic but the patient will also benefit from initial opioid analgesia and/or antispasmodic analgesics before the NSAIDs take effect. Some may need regular opioids or patient-controlled analgesia (PCA).

Antibiotics: Appropriate antibiotics should be prescribed only if you are suspicious that there is co-existing infection because of raised WCC or CRP. This can be either orally with a quinolone or intravenous gentamicin depending on the condition of the patient.

Nephrostomy: When there is attendant pyonephrosis, sepsis and obstruction, it may be necessary to insert a nephrostomy tube. The stone can be removed at a later date when the sepsis has settled.

Treatment of urinary tract stones depends on:

- The symptoms the patient is experiencing
- The effects that the stone is having on renal drainage and therefore function
- The site of the stone as this affects how the stone can be accessed

Treatment should be kept as minimally invasive as possible. Work through the treatments in Table 4.2, asking yourself whether a treatment is appropriate before moving on to the next.

Most stones < 4 mm will pass spontaneously. For stones that do not pass spontaneously (usually > 5 mm) shockwave lithotripsy (ESWL) may be appropriate and, if not, ureteroscopy, ideally with a holmium YAG laser to fragment the stone and appropriate instruments to prevent proximal migration and extract fragments. Percutaneous stone extraction, laparoscopy or open surgery may be required if less invasive treatments fail.

Table 4.2 Treatment options for renal/ureteric stones

Conservative management	OPD review with KUB films usually
Extracorporeal shockwave lithotripsy	Outpatient treatment with > 80% success
Endoscopy via natural orifice (ureteroscopy, cystoscopy, etc)	Effective, but usually requires general anaesthesia
Endoscopy percutaneous nephrolithotomy (PCNL)	1-cm skin incision, but has risks and requires expertise
Endoscopy trans-coelomic laparoscopy	Reserved for large ureteric stones resistant to other forms of management
Open surgery	For large staghorn calculi or large bladder stones

URINARY TRACT INFECTION AND PYELONEPHRITIS

- UTI: $> 10^5$/ml bacteria (or colony-forming units) in urine. Arises due to ascending infection (mostly from faecal flora). Very rarely they are secondary to a bacteraemia
- Simple, recurrent or complicated (abnormal anatomy or foreign body)
- 90% due to Gram-negative bacilli (coliforms) in the community. The others mainly caused by Gram-positive cocci (enterococci)
- More common in females (shorter urethra)
- Common in all age groups

Note: It is common for patients with indwelling urinary catheters to grow *Pseudomonas* in the urine. This is usually due to colonisation and does not require antibiotics unless the urine microscopic examination reveals a bacterial count or WCC that is consistent with infection and the patient is symptomatic.

> **PREDISPOSING FACTORS FOR UTI**
>
> - Urinary obstruction
> - Instrumentation/catheterisation
> - Diabetes
> - Extremes of age
> - Pregnancy
> - Calculi
> - Congenital anomalies
> - Constipation
> - Female

History

- Pain
  - Loin → suprapubic
  - Constant loin pain if pyelonephritis

- Filling symptoms – frequency, dysuria, urgency, nocturia
- Change in smell of urine
- Cloudy urine
- Incontinence
- Retention
- Rigors
- Haematuria
- Vomiting
- Previous episodes
- Past medical history (diabetes mellitus, immunosuppressants, calculi)

It is common to have cystitis associated with pyelonephritis as the infecting bacteria pass from the kidney to the bladder. Cystitis itself should not cause any significant systemic upset. In children it can be very difficult to identify the nature of the UTI as they may not be able to localise the pain. The presence or absence of systemic symptoms can be a great help (Table 4.3).

Table 4.3 Symptoms associated with urinary tract infection

	Lower urinary tract infection (cystitis)	**Upper urinary tract infection (pyelonephritis)**
Pain	Suprapubic	Loin
Filling symptoms	+++	++ or +++
Voiding pain	+++	++ or +++
Smelly urine	+++	++ or +++
Haematuria	+	+
Vomiting/anorexia	−	++
Rigors	−	++
Fever	−	++
Malaise	−	++

Examination

- Temperature and pulse
- Feel for suprapubic and loin tenderness
- Check for systemic sepsis, dehydration and shock
- A catheter may be present

Investigations

- FBC, U&E, CRP, glucose, blood cultures
- Urine dipstick – the presence of nitrites or leukocyte esterase suggests a Gram-negative infection
- Urine microscopy, culture and sensitivity
- KUB to exclude a stone and pyonephrosis (might need urgent nephrostomy insertion), USS renal tract with estimation of residual volume post-micturition
- IVU, cystoscopy not needed in the urgent situation unless there are abnormalities on initial imaging

Treatment

- Fluid resuscitation as required
- Antipyretics
- Treat any underlying predisposing factors

- Antibiotics – base on culture if possible or start with trimethoprim for community-acquired infection or ciprofloxacin if symptomatic. Simple cystitis can be treated with a 3-day course of antibiotics. Recurrent episodes of cystitis require a prolonged (up to 6 months) course. Pyelonephritis more often is associated with nausea, anorexia and vomiting, so may require parenteral antibiotics. Gentamicin in a dose of 5 mg/kg as a single daily infusion is effective against most coliforms, but will require monitoring if more than three doses are given. Pyelonephritis usually requires a 2-week course and treatment of any underlying aetiology. Your hospital will have an antibiotic policy
- Note that a proved UTI in a man requires a renal USS, urinary flow rate measurement and cystoscopy to detect possible anatomical cause. Infection in men may be as a consequence of bladder outlet obstruction

---

UTI IN CHILDREN

- Affects 1% of boys and 3% of girls. Often associated (30%) with vesico-ureteric reflux (also posterior urethral valves, neuropathic bladder and calculi). Reflux can result in parenchymal scarring, hypertension and renal failure
- All neonates and boys require investigation after UTI

HAEMATURIA

This may be macroscopic (15%) or microscopic (85%) (Table 4.4): both require investigation to rule out a malignancy. Macroscopic haematuria occurs in approximately 1% of the population. Microscopic haematuria occurs in 5%. Up to half of patients with haematuria will have an underlying abnormality; 10% of patients with microscopic haematuria and 35% with macroscopic haematuria will go on to be diagnosed with a urological malignancy. Remember the other rarer causes of red urine: rifampicin, myoglobinuria, porphyria and beetroot consumption. Also in female patients, remember to establish that it is true haematuria and not vaginal blood loss.

Table 4.4 Causes of haematuria

Surgical	Malignancy (renal cell or transitional cell carcinoma; also advanced prostate cancer) Traumatic Stone (renal, ureteric, bladder)
Glomerular	IgA nephropathy Glomerulonephritis Systemic lupus erythematosus Embolus
Infective	UTI Tuberculosis Schistosomiasis
Other	Polycystic kidney disease Renal vein thrombosis Vascular malformation Over-anticoagulation Blood dyscrasias/sickle cell disease Exercise-induced haematuria

History

- Acute or chronic
- Associated pain, dysuria, frequency, rigors, weight loss, bone pain

  ○ Painful haematuria likely due to calculus or UTI
  ○ Painless haematuria is suspicious of malignancy

- Timing of haematuria

  ○ Blood at beginning of stream or independent of micturition → urethral source
  ○ Blood at end of stream → bladder origin
  ○ Blood throughout → renal or bladder

- Drug history (warfarin, aspirin, rifampicin)
- Family history (eg polycystic disease)
- Accompanying symptoms – weight loss, bone pain, night sweats, etc
- Foreign travel/swimming in fresh water → schistosomiasis
- Smoking

Examination

- Temperature and pulse rate
- Loin/suprapubic tenderness, masses, palpable kidney
- Rectal examination for prostatic disease in men or pelvic examination in women
- Anaemia
- Cachexia

Note: Menstruation may be confused with haematuria (re-check dipstick after period finished).

Investigations

All patients should have the following:

- Urine dipstick
- MSU for microscopy, culture and sensitivity
- Cytology
- FBC, U&E, coagulation, LFT (PSA in males over 50)
- USS renal tract (good for looking at renal parenchyma) and IVU (good at imaging the urothelium)
- Flexible cystoscopy

Depending on the results of the initial investigations further tests may be required, eg CT abdomen, GA cystoscopy, ureteroscopy or flexible uretero-renoscopy.

Treatment

Definitive treatment dependent upon aetiology. Gross macroscopic haematuria can become complicated by clot retention of urine. This is treated by per-urethral catheterisation, preferably using a three-channel catheter that allows bladder irrigation and washouts to remove the clot. Persistent haematuria may require cystoscopy with washout and cautery.

URINARY RETENTION

Urinary retention is predominantly a condition of elderly men. This may be acute (painful) or chronic (painless). In acute cases, catheterise prior to taking the history as the patient is often in a great deal of pain. Catheterisation is the most effective way of relieving this. Chronic retention (painless) can cause hydronephrosis or renal impairment. Delay catheterisation until you have seen the U&E.

Table 4.5 Causes of urinary retention

Bladder	Bladder calculus Atonic detrusor (postoperatively, anticholinergics, antidepressants) Blood clot
Prostate	Benign prostatic hypertrophy Prostatic carcinoma Prostatitis
Urethra	Stone Stricture Trauma/clot Constipation
Neurological	Spinal injury Lower motor neurone dysfunction Stroke
Other	Constipation Immobility UTI Postoperative abdominal surgery Anal pain

History

- Pain (typically suprapubic) → 500 ml in bladder will cause pain
- When was urine last passed
- Pre-existing outflow obstruction (dribbling, poor flow, hesitancy, nocturia, increased urinary frequency, etc)
- Haematuria
- Weight loss
- Bone pain → malignancy
- Constipation
- Overflow incontinence
- Previous surgery

Examination

- Palpable bladder (if can't feel bladder, carry out an ultrasound scan of bladder to give an idea of bladder volume). If very little urine in bladder and patient isn't passing urine, does the patient have acute renal failure or shock?

- Signs of dehydration
- Always do a rectal examination (prostate, constipation, tone, sensation)

Investigations
- FBC, U&E, glucose
- Bladder USS
- MSU sample

Note: Retention will cause a falsely high PSA.

Treatment
Catheterise (aseptic technique, prophylactic antibiotics as required) and make a note of residual volume. Always re-examine your patient after catheterisation to make sure that the suprapubic mass, pain and tenderness have gone (eg a diverticular abscess can cause all of these and oliguria).

Watch for diuresis and subsequent dehydration if there is evidence of chronic renal impairment or fluid overload (may need iv fluids). If unable to catheterise the urethra, obtain senior help. They may be able to catheterise the patient using a different type of catheter or, if not, a suprapubic catheter will be required. **Do not use a suprapubic catheter if the bladder is impalpable as bowel injury and misplacement is highly likely**. Treat constipation or UTI as required. Irrigation catheter may be needed if retention is secondary to clot.

A trial without catheter (TWOC) can be considered after 24 hours, when the underlying cause has been managed and renal function has normalised. α-Blockers such as tamsulosin or alfuzosin may be considered prior to TWOC.

SCROTAL/TESTICULAR PAIN

This affects all age groups, with testicular torsion of testis/appendage more common in childhood and adolescence, and epididymitis/orchitis more common in men. The latter is commonly caused by *Chlamydia* (younger men) or coliforms (older men).

Inguino-scrotal herniae and varicocele, although usually asymptomatic, can cause vague discomfort. Ten per cent of testicular tumours present with pain.

CAUSES OF TESTICULAR PAIN

- Torsion of testis
- Torsion of testicular appendage
- Trauma
- Epididymo-orchitis (mumps, chlamydia, urinary tract pathogens)
- Ureteric colic – referred pain
- Hernia
- Varicocele
- Tumour – uncommonly presents with pain

History

Patient age is an important determinant of the likely diagnosis. Sudden onset of pain makes torsion more likely, while associated urinary symptoms point to epididymo-orchitis. Especially in cases of torsion, it is important to note the duration of the pain as this can affect whether the testis is likely to be salvageable. It is important to elicit a history of sexually transmitted disease, trauma and a previous history of testicular surgery, maldescent, orchidopexy or previous pains. Long-standing symptoms made worse while standing and in association with swelling suggest a hernia or a varicocele.

Examination

Check for a raised temperature and tachycardia. Tenderness is a feature of orchitis but often the magnitude of pain with torsion precludes examination and can be very well localised particularly with torsion of an appendage. It is important to assess the lie of the testes and palpate for any discrete masses, as there could be a co-existing tumour (rare). It is also important to examine the contralateral testis.

A scrotal swelling is assessed as follows:

- Can you feel above the swelling? If not → hernia
- Is it cystic (fluctuant and traneilluminates)? If so → hydrocoele
- Is there tenderness? If so → epididymo-orchitis, torsion
- Is the testis and epididymis definable?

    ○ If so → epididymo-orchitis, testicular tumour, epididymal cyst
    ○ If not → testicular torsion, hydrocoele

Investigations

- FBC, U&E, MSU and penile/urethral swabs for suspected orchitis
- USS testis with Doppler assessment of the blood supply in experienced hands can be helpful in torsion but should not delay urgent exploration of the testicle if any possibility of torsion

Treatment

- Analgesia and urgent exploration if there is the possibility of torsion
- Quinolone antibiotics for epididymo-orchitis

TESTICULAR TORSION

Testicular torsion is a surgical emergency.

Torsion results in interruption of the blood flow with irreversible injury occurring within 6 hours. Peak incidence is at 10–20 years of age. A high insertion of the tunica vaginalis (the so-called bell clapper testis) makes testicular torsion more likely. This abnormality can be bilateral, hence the need to fix both testicles.

History

- Short onset of severe scrotal pain radiating to lower abdomen
- No urinary symptoms
- May present with abdominal pain (hence the importance of always examining the testicles in males with abdominal pain)
- Up to half may report a previous episode of pain

Examination

- High-riding testicle, very tender to touch, small hydrocoele
- May be associated with pyrexia. Other testicle may lie horizontally (bell-clapper testis)

Investigations

If there is an index of suspicion – call senior urgently as this will need prompt surgical exploration.

Treatment

Urgent surgical exploration. The testicle is retracted out of the scrotal sac via a scrotal incision. Bilateral orchidopexy is performed if the testicle is viable. If the testicle has infarcted then an orchidectomy is carried out. It is important when obtaining consent from these patients to tell them about the risk of testicular loss, and that both testes will be fixed if appropriate. Long-term subfertility may be a problem following fixation.

Torsion of hydatid of Morgagni (testicular appendix)

- Mild to moderate focal pain
- Usually obvious clinically from point tenderness over lateral side of upper pole of testis
- Treatment is conservative, but if there is any suspicion of testicular torsion, the testis should be explored

EPIDIDYMO-ORCHITIS

Acute epididymo-orchitis in older men is usually due to coliform infection arising from the urinary tract, occasionally as a complication of urethral catheterisation, instrumentation or bladder outflow obstruction. In younger men, *Neisseria gonorrhoeae* and *Chlamydia* are the most common pathogens and so a sexual history should be elicited. Full sexual infection screening should be performed in the genito-urinary medicine department as that is better equipped for sampling and contact tracing, etc. Chronic epididymo-orchitis may follow an acute episode or be due to mumps, gonorrhoea or tuberculosis.

History
- Scrotal pain is of slower onset and longer history than torsion
- May have co-existing urinary symptoms
- Penile discharge
- Sexual partners

Examination
- Erythema, swelling and pain overlying testicle with point tenderness over epididymis
- Testicle is not high-riding or as exquisitely tender as in torsion
- May be associated with pyrexia

Investigations
- FBC
- MSU
- Urine for chlamydia polymerase chain reaction (PCR) if appropriate

Treatment
Scrotal support, analgesia and appropriate antibiotics (eg ciprofloxacin for coliforms or doxycycline for suspected chlamydia). On occasion, differentiation from torsion is impossible and requires surgical exploration to establish diagnosis.

VARICOCELE

> Note: Left testicular vein drains into the left renal vein, right testicular vein drains into the inferior vena cava. A new-onset varicocele on the left side occasionally can be a presentation of a left renal tumour.

It is important to remember that varicocele occur due to dilation of the veins within the pampiniform venous plexus (venous drainage of the testis and goes on to form a single testicular vein on each side). Most varicoceles are detected in adolescence/early adulthood; 95% occur on the left side and are idiopathic.

A varicocele feels like a 'bag of worms' within the scrotum and should disappear on lying flat. It rarely requires treatment embolisation is more commonly used than either open or laparoscopic ligation.

IDIOPATHIC SCROTAL OEDEMA

- Usually in boys younger than 10 years
- Presents with an insidious history of pain, redness and oedema
- Testis should feel normal on palpation

TESTICULAR TUMOURS

- Commonest malignancy in young men
- Non-seminomatous germ cell tumours (NSGCT or teratoma) (40%) have a peak incidence at 25 years of age
- Seminoma (50%) peak incidence at 35 years of age
- 5-year survival is 95% if disease is confined to testicle

History

Painless swelling of the body of the testis.

Investigations

- Testicular ultrasound
- CT abdomen
- Serum tumour markers – α-feto protein (AFP), β-human chorionic gonadotrophin (hCG), lactate dehydrogenase (LDH). (AFP produced by yolk sac elements of NSGCT; β-hCG produced by placental-like elements of NSGCT)

Treatment

- Orchidectomy (via inguinal incision)
- Radiotherapy for seminomas
- Platinum-based chemotherapy for NSGCTs

PENILE PROBLEMS

PHIMOSIS

Tight foreskin, which is often due to lichen sclerosis et atrophicus.

History

Often seen in young or arising in childhood. History of balanitis (infection of the foreskin). Ballooning during micturition is normal in young children whose foreskin is still bound down by physiological adhesions.

Treatment

- Depends on age of the patient
- Circumcision may be required, but should be avoided if other options are available

PARAPHIMOSIS

History

Foreskin suffers from moderate phimosis and has been retracted over the glans and will not reduce back over glans so forming a constriction ring. Sometimes after sexual intercourse or urethral instrumentation therefore, always make certain you have replaced the foreskin after catheterisation.

Examination

Pain and swelling of foreskin.

Treatment

- Analgesia, ice pack, topical lidocaine gel prior to manual reduction
- Reduction is a two-handed procedure, with one hand squeezing the glans to reduce the oedema and the other advancing the prepuce over the glans
- Urinary catheter if micturition difficult

- Dorsal slit or circumcision may be required in the acute setting if manual reduction fails – call senior for this
- Discuss elective circumcision at a later date even if the foreskin has been replaced

PRIAPISM

Persistent painful erection lasting > 4 hours. Priapism can be high flow or low flow. Low flow is more common and results from venous stasis and ischaemia. High flow is due to the development of an arterio-cavernosal fistula (often painless).

CAUSES OF PRIAPISM

- Sickle cell disease
- Leukaemia
- Intracavernosal injection
- Pelvic malignancy
- Following penile/spinal cord trauma
- Urogenital inflammation

Early treatment is desirable to prevent future loss of erectile function.

History

- History of trauma/injection
- Blood diseases
- Constitutional illness, weight loss, sweats

Examination

- Glans soft and shaft hard
- Rectal examination – anal tone following trauma, pelvic mass

Treatment

- Involve your seniors
- FBC – look for haemoglobinopathy
- Aspiration and irrigation with heparinised saline
- Check penile blood gases; hypoxia $\rightarrow$ low flow
- Phenylephrine can be injected if aspiration fails

- Drainage procedures into glans, corpora spongiosum or long saphenous vein in low flow have low success rate. Embolisation of arteriovenous malformation in high flow

VASECTOMY

- A segment of the vas deferens is excised with the aim of producing **permanent** sterility, under local or general anaesthetic
- Excised vas should be sent for histological examination to confirm its identity
- Sperm counts at 8 and 12 weeks before abandoning other forms of contraception
- Reasons for failure:

  - Structure other than vas excised
  - Duplex system (ie has two vas on each side)

- Counsel patients about:

  - Irreversibility; reversal operations have variable success rates
  - 1:2000 become fertile again because of recanalisation
  - Takes a while for sperm count to drop
  - Long-term orchialgia in approximately 15%

- Low incidence of haematoma and/or infection

TRAUMA

Ninety per cent of renal trauma is caused by blunt trauma. Nearly half have associated intra-abdominal injury. Yet renal trauma is only present in 10% of cases of abdominal trauma. It is made more likely if there is pre-existing renal abnormality (eg hydronephrosis). Damage to the renal parenchyma is more likely in direct trauma (kidney is squashed against the rib cage). Indirect trauma can result in injury to the vascular pedicle or disruption of the pelviureteric junction.

Do not insert urethral catheters in patients with blood at the external urinary meatus, history of pelvic trauma or high-riding prostate on rectal examination. Involve the urology team.

History
- Timing
- Speed
- Nature of injury

- Seatbelt/passenger/driver/state of vehicle as appropriate
- Associated injuries
- Has any urine passed – has there been any haematuria?

Examination

Remember ATLS principles: Airway, Breathing, Circulation approach

- Look for associated injuries (Note: kidneys can be injured in thoracic trauma!)
- Urine dipstick for haematuria (but a renal pedicle injury is possible with the absence of haematuria)
- Rectal and prostate examination
- Look for blood at the urethral meatus and perineal bruising
- Loin/abdominal abrasions or bruising
- Loin tenderness or mass

Investigations

- All penetrating injuries, macroscopic haematuria, patient with pre-existing renal abnormality, children, microscopic haematuria with systolic BP < 90 mmHg
- CT is the investigation of choice in the stabilised patient (especially if other injuries)
- IVU may be needed in unstable patients to give some information about the unaffected kidney's function

Treatment

- ATLS principles

Eighty per cent are minor (class I/II) and can be treated conservatively. Even grade III and IV injuries may be treated conservatively. Indications for surgery (midline laparotomy) are:

- Uncontrolled haemorrhage
- Associated injuries
- Non-viable parenchyma
- Reno-vascular injuries
- Major urine leak

Renal

> **GRADING**
>
> **I** – contusion (with haematuria)
> **II** – non-expanding subcapsular or perinephric haematoma
> **III** – < 1 cm laceration (no extravasation of urine)
> **iv** – > 1 cm laceration or any laceration extending into the collecting system
> **V** – pedicle injury or completely shattered kidney

Late complications:

- Hypertension
- Hydronephrosis
- Calculi
- Chronic pyelonephritis
- Arteriovenous fistula
- Pseudocyst
- Renal failure

Ureteric

- Mainly penetrating trauma/iatrogenic
- Early signs include haematuria, pain, pyrexia, ileus, U&E derangement
- Later signs are prolonged ileus, obstruction, leakage, anuria, sepsis and fistula
- Imaging – IVU, retrograde ureteropyelography

Bladder

- Mainly due to blunt trauma (especially with full bladder); very often associated with pelvic fracture
- 95% have gross haematuria
- Injury can be either extra- or intra-peritoneal
- Clinical features include suprapubic tenderness and an inability to pass urine
- Investigate with CT or cystogram
- Antibiotic prophylaxis should be given
- Intra-peritoneal rupture requires laparotomy and repair with absorbable sutures and insertion of both urethral and suprapubic catheters

- Extra-peritoneal rupture can be treated conservatively by urethral drainage

Injuries to the bulbar urethra

- Usually secondary to a straddle injury
- May see blood at the meatus and perineal haematoma
- If unable to pass urine, DO NOT pass a urethral catheter as this can convert a partial tear into a complete one. Suprapubic catheter preferable

UROLOGICAL TUMOURS

RENAL CELL CARCINOMA

Renal cell carcinoma (RCC) is longer known as hypernephroma, clear cell tumour or Grawitz tumour.

- Benign kidney tumours are rare. RCC arises from the cells of the proximal tubules. Affects twice as many males as females
- RCC is a cause of 'canon ball' metastases on CXR due to haematological spread
- Sometimes found in hereditary conditions such as von Hippel–Lindau syndrome or familial hereditary papillary cell carcinoma
- Very rare to present with the classic triad of haematuria, loin pain and a loin mass. Can also present as pyrexia of unknown origin and hypertension
- Paraneoplastic syndromes include hypercalcaemia and polycythaemia
- Most found nowadays on USS performed for abdominal pain, ie are incidental findings

Investigations

- Urinalysis, FBC, renal ultrasound, CT abdomen and chest
- May need GFR estimation and renogram for split function

Treatment

- Laparoscopic or open radical nephrectomy
- Partial nephrectomy for small tumours or tumours in a solitary kidney

BLADDER CANCER

- In UK, the majority are transitional cell carcinoma (TCC) (> 90%) with the remainder are either squamous carcinoma or adenocarcinoma
- 80% of TCC are superficial and well differentiated and therefore carry a good prognosis. Occupational exposure to carcinogens such as dyes has become rare due to regulations protecting workers. Smoking is the most common aetiological agent
- Superficial disease can be treated by trans-urethral resection. Regular cystoscopic surveillance is required after surgery. Immunotherapy with intravesical bacille Calmette Guérin (BCG) also of use. Invasive disease needs radical treatment with radiotherapy or cystectomy with some form of urinary diversion

Note: Urothelial tumours can also affect the renal pelvis.

CHAPTER 4

PROSTATE CANCER

- This is the commonest cancer of the male urogenital tract and becomes more common with increasing age (rare before 50). Incidence in the UK is 10 000 cases per year
- 10% of TURP specimens for benign prostatic hyperplasia have adenocarcinoma on histological examination
- All are adenocarcinoma and tend to arise in the posterior part of the gland. Spreads mainly by local invasion through the prostate capsule – lymphatic spread also common. Has a predilection for metastases to bone (especially the vertebral column) due to part of the venous drainage of the prostate draining via a plexus in and around the vertebrae
- Two-third present with symptoms of bladder outflow obstruction
- Rectal examination – may feel prostate enlargement with loss of the central sulcus with or without a palpable nodule

Investigations
- PSA (unlikely if PSA < 10 ng/ml, but benign prostatic hyperplasia (BPH) can cause very high PSA. Similarly, prostate cancer can have low/absent PSA)
- Trans-rectal ultrasound plus biopsy
- Pelvic CT/MRI
- Bone scans if bony metastases suspected

Treatment

Treatment depends on stage of disease and fitness of the patient, ranging from observation to radiotherapy to radical prostatectomy. Hormonal therapy is an essential part of the management armamentarium, eg with goserelin (luteinising hormone-releasing hormone agonist), cyproterone acetate (anti-androgen).

URINARY INCONTINENCE

There are several types of urinary incontinence.

- **Stress** (leaks when laughing, coughing, etc): most often secondary to pelvic floor trauma during childbirth. Treat with pelvic floor exercises and physiotherapy in the first instance. May need surgery
- **Urge** (involuntary urinary loss due to detrusor overactivity): causes include idiopathic detrusor overactivity, neuropathy or secondary to an intravesical irritative lesion, eg UTI or bladder stone. Exclude a serious cause. Bladder 're-training' can be used in combination with such drugs as anticholinergics to depress detrusor activity
- **Mixed**: mixture of stress and urge
- **Overflow**: occurs because of bladder distension secondary to bladder outlet obstruction, detrusor atony, neurologic impairment of the bladder. Sometimes requires long-term catheterisation or intermittent catheterisation

Table 4.6 Causes of urinary incontinence

Infective	UTI
Neurological	Cerebrovascular accident
	Dementia
	Brain tumours
	Parkinsonism
	Multiple sclerosis
	Pelvic floor injury
	Iatrogenic injury to pelvic nerves
	Spinal cord compression/injury/tumour, etc
	Detrusor overactivity
Mechanical	Bladder outflow obstruction (overflow)

History

- Childbirth
- Pelvic/urological surgery
- Pain
- When does the patient leak? Do they have the desire to void? Can they control it?
- Neurological symptoms
- Past medical history
- Drug history
- Frequency, urgency, nocturia, etc

Investigations

- MSU, microscopy and culture
- U&E
- Lateral cystogram
- USS – pre- and post-micturition volumes
- Voiding diary
- Cystometrogram (looks at detrusor pressure during filling and during urinary flow)
- Cysto-urethroscopy

Treatment

- Treat cause
- Pelvic floor exercises are useful in both stress and urge incontinence (strong contractions of the pelvic floor muscles can inhibit detrusor activity thereby helping with urge incontinence)
- Vaginal weights
- Lifestyle modification – avoid large volumes of fluid before bedtime, avoid excessive caffeine, etc
- Bladder training
- Electrical training and biofeedback
- Drugs – anticholinergics (eg oxybutynin or toltcrodine), NOT if history of glaucoma

(See also Chapter 2, page 91.)

This is a synergistic, bacterial, necrotising fasciitis that affects the perineum, genital and perianal areas. It spreads rapidly along fascial planes, stripping the skin of its blood supply, and requires emergency resuscitation, extensive debridement and appropriate antibiotics. It can spread very, very quickly leading to systemic sepsis, shock and eventual multiorgan failure and death. Multiple debridements are often required and it is a good idea to have another look after 24 hours under GA to both change the dressings and debride any further necrotic tissue.

The testicles are rarely involved as they have a separate blood supply to the affected region. The source of the sepsis can be anorectal (eg perianal abscess, perforated rectum), urological (instrumentation, epididymitis) or cutaneous. Advancing age, alcohol misuse and diabetes are often present.

Early on in the disease, there is often little to find aside from tenderness. As the disease progresses, discoloration, subcutaneous crepitations and gangrene ensue. Pain is out of proportion to the initial findings perianally, this may subside as necrosis spreads to involve nerve tissue. The skin appearance (may be a very small patch of necrosis) underestimates the degree of underlying disease.

CHAPTER 5

TRAUMA AND ORTHOPAEDICS

G E COLGAN AND J P MCELWAIN

TOPICS

The basic principles of fracture management are applicable to nearly every type of fracture regardless of site or severity. Extensive knowledge of the technicalities of orthopaedic surgery is not necessary to properly assess and manage an injured patient. Try to develop a comprehensive method of assessing a patient with isolated or multiple injuries. This will make your examination efficient and you will be less likely to miss anything. No amount of knowledge replaces a thorough examination of joints, soft tissues, neurovascular status and loss of function. It is important to be aware of certain patterns of injury, and the possibility of other associated injuries. If you know about them, you will automatically look for them.

A fracture is defined as any breach in the cortex of a bone. Fractures may be **simple** (two main bone fragments) or **comminuted** (three or more fragments), sometimes referred to as multifragmentary. Comminuted fractures usually involve higher energy. Fractures may be open or closed – depending on the soft tissue continuity over the injured bone. Fractures can be caused by direct trauma, ie a direct blow, or indirectly by a twisting or bending injury.

Pathological fractures can occur with minimal force, or in the absence of trauma in a diseased or abnormal bone. Examples of pathological fractures include osteoporosis, Paget's disease, primary or secondary tumours of bone. Avulsion fractures occur when a ligament shears off a small fragment of bone at its attachment. Crush fractures occur from compression forces such as a fall from a height.

If you are seeing a patient in Accident and Emergency (A&E) with a fracture, the question you need to ask is: does this need an immediate orthopaedic assessment or can the patient be seen in the fracture clinic? Any fracture which is angulated, displaced or rotated (Table 5.1, Figure 5.1) may require surgical reduction and/or fixation, and should be discussed with the orthopaedic surgeons if you are unsure. The fracture clinic is devised to follow-up patients who do not require admission for surgery. Essentially, a patient with an undisplaced fracture, not involving a joint or major long bone, with no open wound, or neurovascular deficit can be treated in A&E with a splint or cast, and referred to the clinic after adequate assessment. If in doubt, seek an orthopaedic opinion. See Table 5.2 for how to describe a fracture.

Table 5.1 Fractures: basic terms and how to assess

Displacement	• Refers to loss of alignment of the fractured bone. It is caused by the deforming trauma of the injury, or by the unopposed contraction of muscles attached to the fracture fragments • If there is no deformity the fracture is said to be undisplaced • Displacement is described as the position of the distal fragment relative to the proximal fragment • Normally the amount (as a percentage) and direction of displacement is described, eg 75% lateral displacement • Displacement should be assessed for on both AP and lateral X-rays
Angulation	• Refers to the tilting of the fracture itself • This can cause confusion, so it is easier to describe the angulation of the distal fragment relative to the proximal fragment • The direction and amount of angulation (expressed in degrees) is described, ie the distal fragment has 30° medial angulation • Angulation should be assessed for on both AP and lateral X-rays
Rotation	• Rotation occurs when the distal fracture fragment 'twists' relative to the proximal fragment • Can be difficult to appreciate on an X-ray, and is usually assessed clinically • Metacarpal and phalangeal fractures should all be assessed for a rotational deformity. This is done by assessing the position of the fingers relative to each other in metacarpophalangeal (MCP) joint flexion

Figure 5.1 Diagrammatic illustration of displacement, angulation and rotation

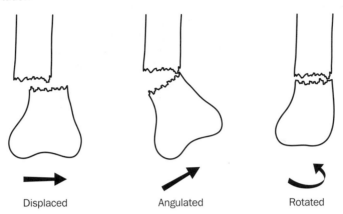

Displaced   Angulated   Rotated

Table 5.2 Describing a fracture

Anatomical location	Name of the bone or bones involved
Site on the bone	Epiphysis Diaphyseal/shaft Metaphyseal Physis/growth plate for skeletally immature patients Intra-articular/extra-articular
Fracture type	Simple/comminuted Open/closed Pathological/avulsion/crush

Shape of fracture	Simple:
	   Spiral
	   Oblique
	   Transverse
	
	Comminuted:
	   Three-part fracture with butterfly fragment
	   Segmental
	   Multifragmentary

CHAPTER 5

189

GENERAL MANAGEMENT OF FRACTURES

History

The mechanism of injury should be carefully elicited – whether it is a road traffic accident, fall or assault, or the absence of trauma. This will help you assess the likely forces that caused injury and the possibility of pathological fractures or associated injuries. Relevant medical/surgical history and tetanus status are important to assess. It is essential to ask about occupation and hand dominance when assessing injuries, particularly of the upper limb.

Examination

- Advanced Trauma Life Support (ATLS) protocol examination is ideal for trauma patients and should not be omitted, regardless of injury
- Fracture site and the position should be noted with any gross deformity or skin/soft tissue damage
- Peripheral blood supply/pulses/capillary refill/peripheral temperature should be documented and acted on if compromised
- The neurological status should be assessed by examining motor/sensation/reflexes
- For limb injuries, particularly the lower limb, it is essential to assess for compartment syndrome (see pages 219–220).

Investigations

If a fracture is suspected two X-rays taken in two planes at 90° to one another should be obtained (anteroposterior (AP) and lateral views) (Table 5.3). It is a tradition in the case of fractures of the long bones to include the joint above and below the injury site. Retake X-rays if it is necessary to achieve this. It may be necessary to reduce and splint a grossly deformed limb or displaced fracture prior to X-ray, such as an ankle dislocation with ischaemic foot or femoral shaft fracture. In this case, the reduction should be carried out first, and a temporary splint or back slab applied. X-rays can be obtained through the splint/slab. When there is co-morbidity or significant injury, or the patient requires surgery, bloods should be taken for FBC, renal function, coagulation screen and blood crossmatched.

Table 5.3 Fracture patterns

Cervical spine	5% of patients with a cervical spine injury have another cervical spine fracture at a different level (contiguous injury)
Thoracolumbar spine	Any patient with one vertebral fracture should have full imaging of the C-, T- and L-spine as 5–10% will have another fracture elsewhere in the spine (non-contiguous injury)
Shoulder injury	Patients with shoulder pain following a fall should have an AP and lateral axillary view to rule-out a posterior dislocation
Ulnar shaft	Isolated ulnar shaft fracture on forearm: X-ray will need imaging of the proximal radio-ulnar joint to check for elbow dislocation – Monteggia's fracture
Radial shaft	Isolated radial shaft fracture on forearm: X-ray will need imaging of the distal radio-ulnar joint to check for wrist dislocation Galeazzi's fracture
Pelvis	The pelvis is a solid ring and usually fractures in two places so if you see one fracture in the pelvis look for another often diagonally opposite the diagnosed fracture
Femoral shaft	Always image the joint above and below the fracture as ipsilateral hip fractures are missed, particularly in middle-third shaft fractures. Rule-out ipsilateral proximal tibial fractures
Knee dislocations	Assume vascular injury with a knee dislocation, even if pulses present (often intimal tear that extends with time). Patients require urgent reduction and vascular assessment ± angiography

continued

Table 5.3 *Continued*

Fibula	Mid-shaft fibular fractures are 'high Weber C' fractures and can be associated with syndesmosis injuries – need mortise ankle view
Medial malleolus	An isolated medial malleolus fracture on X-ray is often associated with a missed fracture of the proximal fibular neck, and/or syndesmosis injuries – Maisonneuve's fracture
Ankle	Syndesmosis injuries are seen in Weber C type fractures, but may not be obvious on AP X-ray. Mortise view to assess talar shift
Calcaneus	Up to 10% of calcaneus fractures are associated with a lumbar spine injury. Assess $\pm$ X-ray lumbar spine

TREATMENT

Careful attention should be paid to airway and breathing with supplemental oxygen. It is sensible to attain iv access as trauma or long-bone fractures can often involve significant blood loss. In young people often the only sign of significant hypovolaemia is tachycardia so iv fluids should be started. It is unacceptable to allow patients to be in pain, and analgesia should be titrated until the patient is pain free before X-ray. See also Table 5.4.

Table 5.4 General principles of management of fractures

Assess	Neurovascular assessment
Reduce	Align the fracture by correcting significant deformity
Wound management	See section on open fractures, pages 198–200
Immobilisation	Thick back-slab – generally immobilises the joint above and below to prevent displacement
Reassess	Reassess neurovascular status after reduction + splinting

The ATLS guidelines are a comprehensive system for assessing the multiply injured patient. The priority in trauma is to save life then limb (Table 5.5). The initial aim is to secure a protected airway, oxygenate the patient, and restore circulating volume (see Tables 5.6 and 5.7) using the primary survey. In general the '**rule of 3s**' applies: 3 ml of iv fluid should be given for every 1 ml of blood lost.

Orthopaedic injuries are rarely immediately life-threatening as massive haemorrhage is usually due to intra-thoracic or intra-abdominal injury but it can be due to major amputations or severe pelvic fractures. Any bleeding from a limb should be controlled by direct pressure where possible.

Table 5.5 General management of the patient with multiple trauma

PRIMARY SURVEY	AIRWAY, BREATHING AND CIRCULATORY PROBLEMS
Airway	Assess and protect airway, oxygenate patient while maintaining cervical spine protection. Intubate if required
Breathing	Auscultate lungs. Identify and treat pneumothorax/tension pneumothorax at this stage
Circulation	Assess BP and pulse (see also Tables 5.6 and 5.7). Direct pressure to bleeding sites
	Large bore iv access; iv fluids – 2 litres Hartmann's STAT ± blood replacement
Disability	Determine level of consciousness, Glasgow Coma Scale score and pupil reactivity
Environment	Expose patient fully. Prevent hypothermia

continued

CHAPTER 5

Table 5.5 *Continued*

INITIAL MANAGEMENT	
Trauma X-rays	Lateral cervical spine, CXR, AP pelvis
Intravenous access	Large bore iv × 2 antecubital veins
Bloods	FBC, U&E, LFT, coagulation, amylase, glucose, toxicology screen and crossmatch as required. ABG
Fluid resuscitation	2 litres Hartmann's STAT – blood products as required
Analgesia	Conscious patients with multiple injuries require iv opioid analgesia
Reassess	Reassess ABCs to see if patient stabilising with these measures – rapid/transient/non-responder?
SECONDARY SURVEY	**HEAD-TO-TOE EXAMINATION TO IDENTIFY OTHER INJURIES**
Limb injuries	Try to reduce and splint any grossly deformed limb. Dress open wounds. Identify limb-threatening injuries
	If ABCs stable – X-ray of suspected injuries
	If unstable – ABCs must take priority
Further imaging	CT, etc may be required depending on stability and injuries of the patient. Unstable patients require emergency surgery/management, not lengthy diagnostic tests

The secondary survey is used to identify most orthopaedic injuries. Large bone fractures are more obvious injuries, and should be easily detected during assessment of the limbs. Smaller injuries are easily missed, particularly in the unstable young trauma patient, when the focus is on the more urgent life-threatening injuries. In the immediate situation a hand or finger injury may seem an insignificant fracture, but it can lead to lifelong disability when the patient recovers from the initial trauma, if it is not detected early and treated appropriately.

Table 5.6 Blood loss from fractures

Blood loss (ml)	% Blood loss	BP	Pulse (beats/min)	Respiratory rate (breaths/min)	Treatment
> 750	1–15	Normal	< 100	14–20	Fluid
750–1500	15–30	Normal	> 100	20–30	Fluid
1500–2500	30–40	↓	> 120	30–40	Fluid and blood
> 2500	> 40	↓	> 140	> 35	Fluid and blood

Table 5.7 Potential blood loss from specific fractures

Fracture	Laterality	Blood loss (ml)	% Blood loss	Class of shock
Pelvis	–	Potentially several litres	Up to 100	I–IV
Humerus	Unilateral	750	15	I–II
Tibia	Unilateral	750	15	I–II
	Bilateral	1500	30	II–III
Femur	Unilateral	1500	30	II–III
	Bilateral	3000	> 40	III–IV

PRIORITIES IN MANAGEMENT

Life-threatening injuries

PRIMARY SURVEY

A Airway and cervical spine protection
B Breathing
C Circulation – with haemorrhage control
D Disability
E Environment/exposure

Patients should be log rolled with full spinal precautions

Use the primary survey to identify and treat all life-threatening injuries – airway obstruction, chest injuries, haemorrhage, before assessing the patient for fractures (Table 5.5). Do not delay urgent life-saving treatment while obtaining large numbers of X-rays in the A&E department! (You can do this in the operating theatre if necessary when the patient is anaesthetised.)

Limb-threatening

Following the primary survey, a complete examination from head to toe is undertaken – the secondary survey (Table 5.5 and box below). All major orthopaedic injuries should be identified during this stage and treated along the guidelines for specific fracture management.

SECONDARY SURVEY

Head and face

- Inspect pupils for reactivity/equality and eye injuries
- Ears for haemotympanum or cerebrospinal fluid (CSF) leaks
- Face for facial bone injuries or lacerations
- Mouth for dental alignment, lacerations
- Palpate scalp for contusions, lacerations or fractures

Neck and cervical spine

- Inspect venous distension
- Subcutaneous emphysema
- Palpate C-spine tenderness in conscious, alert patient
- Bony alignment/deformity
- Tracheal deviation

Chest wall

- Inspect penetrating injury, asymmetrical movements, bruising
- Palpate for rib fractures, subcutaneous emphysema, tenderness
- Auscultate for breath sounds – present/symmetrical
- Heart sounds
- Percuss for resonance/dullness; compare both sides

SECONDARY SURVEY

(*continued*)

Abdomen

- Inspect wounds, bruising, movement with respiration
- Palpate for tenderness, masses, guarding, pregnancy
- Auscultate for bowel sounds
- Percuss for subtle tenderness, perforation

Pelvis/perineum

- Inspect external genitalia – bruising, lacerations, blood at penile meatus
- Palpate testis for rupture, scrotal haematoma; avoid compressing/distracting the pelvis
- Rectal examination – blood, open pelvic injury, sphincter tone, high riding prostate, perianal/saddle sensation
- Vaginal examination – blood, open pelvic injury

Upper limbs

- Look for deformity, bruises, lacerations
- Feel – crepitus/tenderness along the length of arm, forearm, wrist, hand and each digit, pulses – radial, ulnar and brachial; compare sides
- Move – examine the range of motion in shoulder, elbow, wrist and finger joints (active movement in conscious patient, passive in unconscious)
- Neurological examination – sensation (all dermatomes C5–T1)
- Reflexes – biceps (C5/6), triceps (C7/8) and brachioradialis (C5/6) (supinator)
- Power and tone – assess in conscious patient

Lower limbs

- Look for deformity, bruises, lacerations
- Feel – crepitus/tenderness along the length of thigh, leg, foot and toes
- Feel – pulses (femoral, popliteal, post. tibial and dorsalis pedis); compare sides

continued

- Move – examine the range of motion in hip, knee ankle and foot (active movement in conscious patient, passive in unconscious)
- Neurological examination – sensation (all dermatomes L1–S2)
- Reflexes – knee (L3/4), ankle (S1/2), plantar (S1/2)
- Power and tone – assess in conscious patient

Spinal assessment

- Inspect – lacerations, bruising, deformity
- Palpate – thoraco-lumbar spine for tenderness, step deformity
- Neurological exam – check peripheral tone, power, co-ordination, sensation reflexes; rectal examination for anal tone

Disability-threatening

Definitive fixation of non-limb-threatening fractures may have to be deferred until the patient is more stable. The priority is to stabilise the patient and treat injuries that are more serious first. However, even smaller injuries need to be identified and treated appropriately as soon as possible, as they can lead to significant morbidity once the patient has recovered.

OPEN FRACTURES

These are fractures with part of the bone exposed to the external environment. In general, the greater the soft tissue injury, the greater the force imparted in causing the fracture. Proper management of the soft tissue injury is vital to a good functional outcome.

These wounds can be described as either 'in-out', where the fracture fragment pierces the skin, or 'out-in' wounds, where the skin is breached by an external object or force resulting in fracture. 'Out-in' wounds are more contaminated, and have a higher rate of infection.

Soft tissue injury is described by Gustilo and Anderson's classification (Table 5.8), but often the extent of soft tissue injury cannot be appreciated until the patient is in theatre, so the grading may be falsely low in A&E.

Table 5.8 Gustilo and Anderson's classification of fractures

Type	Description	Antibiotic
1	Small < 1 cm, clean wound. Minimal injury to soft tissue and periosteum	First-generation cephalosporin
2	> 1 cm wound, but no significant soft tissue damage/periosteal stripping, flaps or avulsions	First-generation cephalosporin
3 (a–c)	Larger wounds, but more importantly – extensive injury to muscle periosteum and bone. Farmyard injuries* and gunshot wounds are in this category:	
	3 (a) Extensive contamination or injury, but adequate soft tissue to cover bone	First-generation cephalosporin + aminoglycoside
	3 (b) Extensive injury to soft tissue, usually requiring soft tissue transfer for coverage	First-generation cephalosporin + aminoglycoside + penicillin
	3 (c) Open fractures with a neurovascular injury necessitating repair	
* Farmyard injuries should also be treated with iv metronidazole for anaerobic cover.		

History

- Last meal
- Mechanism, location and time of injury
- Tetanus status and allergies
- Pertinent medical history

Examination

- ATLS standard assessment to rule-out other injuries including complete exposure and assessment of the injured limb
- It is important to assess circulation of the affected limb by examination of peripheral pulses, capillary refill, temperature distal limb and Doppler USS if necessary
- Sensation – check all dermatomes
- Movement distal to fracture – joints/digits
- Assess for any sign of compartment syndrome

Investigations

- Bloods – FBC, U&E, coagulation, group and save, crossmatch (depending on site of fracture)
- Two X-rays at right angles to each other including the joint above and below, ie AP + lateral views
- CXR if indicated for anaesthetic

Treatment

- Intravenous access – large bore $\times$ 2
- Keep fasting as these patients generally need to go to theatre urgently
- Intravenous fluids – amount depending on blood loss and site of fracture
- Intravenous analgesia – Cyclimorph (morphine tartrate and cyclizine tartrate)/morphine titrated to achieve adequate analgesia; these patients need plenty of pain relief
- Tetanus toxoid/immunoglobulins – depends on tetanus status of patient, but usually indicated
- Antibiotic prophylaxis – see Table 5.8
- Wound swab (not very useful, but should be taken prior to antibiotics)
- Wound management – remove any gross contaminants, and irrigate with sterile water. Take a Polaroid photo of wound – provides a record and prevents unnecessary repeat tampering with wound!
- Cover the wound with sterile dressings. Align the limb and splint in thick back-slab
- Reassess neurovascular status after fracture splinting
- Urgent orthopaedic review

Remember: Compartment syndrome does occur in open fractures. The limb is not decompressed because of the open injury, and in fact as open fractures are often associated with a higher energy trauma, compartment syndrome is more likely to occur! See page 219.

Hip fractures are extremely common orthopaedic injuries, and their treatment in A&E should be standard. Often these are elderly patients with co-morbid medical conditions. These patients should have a full medical assessment to identify or pre-empt any conditions that may delay surgery. An elderly patient may have been on a cold floor for hours – leading to dehydration, hypothermia, etc. Also, exclude a medical cause for the patient falling in the first place. Morbidity and mortality increase with surgery after 24 hours, so any medical problems should be recognised and dealt with promptly.

A young patient with an intra-capsular hip fracture (Figure 5.2) is an orthopaedic emergency as they are at risk of avascular necrosis of the femoral head. Ideally the patient should be operated on within 6 hours from the time of injury. Any elderly patient who has a history of falls who is complaining of hip pain and is unable to weight bear has a hip fracture until proved otherwise. Even if the X-ray shows no obvious fracture, these patients should be admitted, as often they have an impacted fracture that is not obvious on the initial X-ray. Further imaging or repeated plain X-rays are required for further investigation.

Figure 5.2 Garden's classification of intra-capsular hip fractures

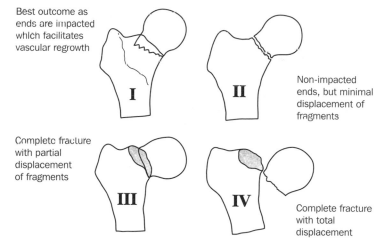

Best outcome as ends are impacted which facilitates vascular regrowth

I

II

Non-impacted ends, but minimal displacement of fragments

Complete fracture with partial displacement of fragments

III

IV

Complete fracture with total displacement

Inter-trochanteric hip fractures are extra-capsular, and there is no compromise to the blood supply to the femoral head. They are usually treated with a dynamic hip screw or short intramedullary nail, depending on the surgeon's preference. Some fractures are at the borderline between being extra-capsular and inter-trochanteric and are usually called basal cervical fractures, ie they occur at the base of the femoral neck. These are usually treated as inter-trochanteric fractures, but this will be decided by the orthopaedic team that reviews the X-rays.

History

- Mechanism and time of injury (not time of arrival in A&E) – fall etc.
- Other injuries – particularly in younger patients. Elderly patient – think head injury, ipsilateral shoulder/wrist fracture
- Any precipitating factors to fall? Chest pain, shortness of breath, syncope,
- Full medical history, co-morbid medical conditions
- Medications/allergies
- Anticoagulants in elderly – may delay spinal anaesthesia

Examination

- Vital signs
- Position of injured limb – usually shortened, externally rotated, flexed at knee and abducted
- Check range of motion gently after the X-ray
- Neurovascular examination – check peripheral pulses, sensation and power to distal limb
- Full medical assessment to rule-out cardiovascular cause for fall and to identify any medical issue that may delay surgery, eg lower respiratory tract infection, etc

Investigations

- Bloods – FBC, U&E, coagulation, group and save (Dynamic Hip Screw)/crossmatch 2 units (hemiarthroplasty)
- CXR, ECG to assess cardiorespiratory fitness
- X-rays – AP pelvis + lateral hip X-ray (may need to X-ray full femur to exclude distal fracture)

Treatment

- Oxygen as required
- Intravenous access large bore × 2
- Intravenous fluids – rehydrate if required and maintenance fluids if fasting overnight
- Opioid analgesia until pain free, and as required
- Early anaesthetic assessment with regard to fitness for surgery
- See also Table 5.9

Table 5.9 Management of intra-capsular hip fractures

X-ray		Treatment		
Class	Displacement	Young patient	Fit elderly patient	Frail elderly patient
I – incomplete fracture (one cortex)	None	DHS	DHS	DHS
II – complete fracture (both cortices)	None	DHS	DHS	DHS
III – complete fracture	Incomplete	DHS	Bipolar hemiarthroplasty	Unipolar hemiarthroplasty
IV – complete fracture	Complete	DHS	Bipolar hemiarthroplasty	Unipolar hemiarthroplasty

PELVIC FRACTURES

The pelvis is a solid ring and disruption at one point, such as an isolated pubic ramus fracture, does not result in mechanical instability. However, fractures at two points on the ring can produce instability. The pelvis may be unstable in two planes: (a) horizontal (and rotationally unstable) and (b) vertical (Figure 5.3). The so-called open-book fracture is an example of the horizontally unstable pelvis and occurs from an AP compression type injury, ie straddle injury or head-on collision into steering column.

Figure 5.3 Pelvic fractures: horizontal and vertical instability

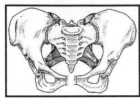

Horizontal instability + external rotation
AP compression forces disrupt the pubic symphysis and the anterior sacroiliac joints. The pelvis opens from the front (the 'open-book' pelvic injury) and both hemipelvises rotate externally. This is unstable in the horizontal plane

Horizontal instability + internal rotation
Lateral compression-type injury caused by a side impact. There is a fracture of the left pubic rami and ipsilateral sacroiliac joint. The left hemipelvis has been compressed or closed and rotated inwards. It is also unstable horizontally

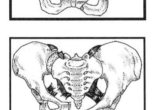

Vertical instability
There is a fracture through the pubic symphysis and right sacroiliac joint with superior displacement of the right hemipelvis. The plane of instability is vertical

History and examination

The forces involved open and externally rotate the hemipelvis. These fractures are often associated with urethral injuries, which must be excluded. Vertically unstable injuries, ie vertical shear injuries, occur from asymmetrical limb loading, for example fall from a height. The patient will often have a leg length discrepancy as the hemipelvis is displaced superiorly relative to the other side.

Disruption of bone fragments that occurs at the time of impact damages the extensive network of blood vessels (usually the venous plexus) within the pelvis and can result in severe haemorrhage.

Clinical assessment of stability by compressing and distracting the iliac wings is not sensitive, and should be avoided as it may dislodge any clots that have already formed. Rectal examination is mandatory to assess for blood, high-riding prostate or potentially open fractures.

Vaginal examination should be performed in female patients as a pelvic fracture can 'open' into the rectum or vagina, and is associated with high level of infection/morbidity and mortality of 30–50%.

Investigations

An AP pelvis X-ray is a much better way to assess a pelvic injury. Pelvic injuries often occur in the multiply traumatised patient, and can be a life-threatening cause of haemorrhage. Pelvis X-ray should be taken early in the resuscitation phase to identify and treat an unstable fracture. Further imaging depends on stability of patient with regard to the appropriateness of DPL (diagnostic peritoneal lavage), CT or surgery. You should always exclude a urethral injury in a male patient with a pelvic injury before catheterisation. A retrograde urethrogram is required, or if this is not available suprapubic catheterisation should be done.

Treatment

- ATLS assessment to identify and treat life-threatening injuries
- Resuscitation with fluid ± blood as per ATLS guidelines
- Reduce the leg length discrepancy in vertically unstable fractures with gentle downward traction on the shortened limb
- Fashion a pelvic sling by tying a sheet tightly around the level of greater trochanters with legs in internal rotation (or using a pelvic sling)
- **Urgent orthopaedic review**
- See Table 5.10

Table 5.10 Management and assessment of pelvic fractures

Mechanical	Haemodynamic	Treatment
Stable	Stable	No specific emergency treatment
Stable	Unstable	Not pelvic bleeding look for source
Unstable	Stable	No urgent treatment of pelvis needed
Unstable	Unstable	Urgent pelvis stabilisation + look for other sources of bleeding

DISTAL RADIAL FRACTURES

Fractures of the distal radius are the commonest fractures in people over the age if 40. They usually follow a fall on an outstretched hand (FOOSH). A young person with a distal radius fracture with displacement or angulation requires treatment. A greater degree of deformity may be acceptable in an elderly frail patient. If the fracture is undisplaced no manipulation is required. As not all distal radial fractures require surgery, or orthopaedic assessment at the time of injury, many can be followed up in the fracture clinic, but the ability to interpret an X-ray of a patient with a distal radial fracture depends on knowledge of the normal anatomy of the wrist. Grossly displaced or angulated fractures can cause compression of the median nerve – acute carpal tunnel syndrome – which may require urgent fracture reduction ± surgical decompression.

History

- Mechanism of injury – FOOSH, standing height or fall from a height?
- Hand dominance and occupation – assess functional demand, is the patient self-employed?
- Past medical/surgical history – are they fit for surgery?
- Medications and allergies

Examination

- Look – deformity. Check skin for puncture wounds
- Feel – palpate pulses. Check capillary refill
- Move – range of movement will be decreased
- Test – assess finger movement + sensation (in particular median nerve)

Investigations

- Bloods – FBC, U&E if for surgery
- CXR + ECG as indicated
- AP X-ray – to identify a fracture of the distal radius. Does it involve the joint? Is it comminuted? Is there a fracture of the ulnar styloid? Normally the radial styloid is about 1 cm longer than the ulnar styloid, and the radial inclination is 22° (angle between the radial styloid and the horizontal) (Figure 5.4). Look for evidence of radial shortening by comparing the relative lengths of the ulnar and radial styloids

Figure 5.4 AP view of distal radius and ulna

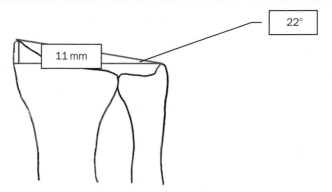

- Lateral X-ray – normally there is an 11° volar/anterior tilt of the distal radial joint surface. Look for evidence of fracture. Is the fracture impacted? Look also for angulation of the fracture – dorsal angulation in Colles-type fracture. Is the distal fragment displaced from the shaft of the radius? Dorsal displacement – Colles-type fracture; volar displacement – Smith's-type fracture

Treatment

- Below-elbow back-slab should be applied and the arm elevated
- Intramuscular analgesia titrated to pain

WRIST FRACTURES REQUIRING MANIPULATION ± FIXATION

- Comminuted fractures
- Intra-articular fracture with > 2 mm step
- Radio-ulnar shortening > 2 mm
- Dorsal displacement
- Dorsal angulation if posterior tilt beyond neutral
- All fractures with volar displacement (Smith's-type fractures)

ANKLE FRACTURES AND DISLOCATIONS

Ankle fractures are common injuries, and deciding which fractures need surgery (open reduction internal fixation), and which fractures are suitable for conservative management can be difficult as some injuries are subtle – 1-mm lateral shift of the talus in the ankle mortise reduces the contact area by 42%! There are certain patterns of injuries in the ankle, and this can be helpful when viewing the X-rays, as you will learn to look specifically for the associated injuries. As with other fractures, an ankle fracture that is undisplaced, with no neurovascular deficit and no significant soft tissue damage, can be treated conservatively with a below-knee back-slab and referred to the next fracture clinic.

A dislocated or subluxated ankle should be considered an orthopaedic emergency, as the vascular supply of the foot may be compromised and sustained stretching or tenting of the skin over the ankle joint (usually the medial malleolus) leads to ischaemia, pressure necrosis and skin breakdown. There is usually an obvious clinical deformity in these cases, and this should be dealt with by prompt reduction under sedation/analgesia and splinting in back-slab **before** taking an X-ray. Waiting for an X-ray to confirm a clinically obvious, grossly deformed ankle will lead to significant delay in fracture reduction.

History

- Mechanism of injury – fall, jumping from a height, road traffic accident, etc?
- Try to ascertain the position of the foot and ankle at the time of injury – supination (inversion)/pronation (eversion). Did the foot rotate, etc?
- Other injuries
- Relevant medical history
- Medications and allergies

Examination

- Look – position of ankle, overlying skin:

  - Is it taut/tented? Open wound?
  - Swelling/bruising ecchymosis

- Feel – tenderness or crepitus over the medial and lateral malleoli. Palpate the ligaments for tenderness. Palpate pulses and test distal sensation and movement

- Move – movements will be decreased in all ankle fractures. Don't forget to assess Achilles' tendon – palpate it directly to feel that it is intact. Test plantar flexion (Thompson's test) – foot should be plantar flexed slightly when the calf is squeezed. It is performed with the patient prone

Investigations

Three X-ray views should be taken for all ankle fractures – AP, lateral and mortise view (the foot is internally rotated 15°, it allows 'head-on' view of the ankle joint).

AP view

Look at the lateral and medial malleolus for fractures. Is there displacement? Look at the overlap of the tibia on the fibula. It should be 5 mm or one-third the width of the fibula. Widening suggests syndesmosis injury, or fracture displacement. The fibula is longer than the medial malleolus and the talocrural angle should be $83 \pm 4°$.

Mortise view

Look at the space around the medial, superior and lateral border of the talus relative to the medial malleolus, distal tibia and lateral malleolus, respectively. Is there even spacing or is the medial clear space widened? This suggests lateral talar shift, ie subluxation due to syndesmosis injury or fracture displacement.

Lateral view

Look for displacement of the fibular fracture ± shortening. Look for posterior malleolus fracture of distal tibia. Look at the congruency of the distal tibia. Bloods should be taken for those patients requiring surgery.

Treatment

All ankle fractures should be placed in a below-knee back-slab and elevated. Classification of ankle fractures is based on the degree of injury to the lateral malleolus (Table 5.11 and Figure 5.5).

Table 5.11 Ankle fractures

Weber A	Fibular fracture below syndesmosis Usually undisplaced and often isolated injuries
Weber B	Fibular fracture at syndesmosis Most likely to be associated with medial malleolar fractures – bimalleolar fracture
Weber C	Fibular fracture above syndesmosis (can include fibular neck fracture – Maisonneuve injury) High incidence of syndesmosis injury ~70%

Figure 5.5 Weber's classification of ankle fractures

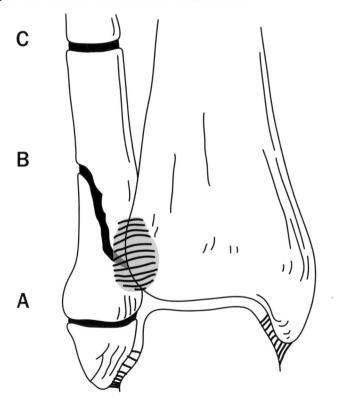

Isolated lateral malleolus fracture

If undisplaced – below-knee back-slab and fracture clinic (usually Weber A). Fixation is indicated if there is:

- A 2-mm displacement or shortening (usually Weber B)
- Talar shift (Weber B + C)
- Syndesmosis injury (usually Weber C)
- Open injury

Isolated medial malleolus fracture

Unless completely undisplaced – usually all these fractures need fixation as there is often soft tissue caught in the fracture site (soft tissue interposition) and these fractures do not heal if treated conservatively.

Bimalleolar fractures

These are very unstable fractures and generally all need to be fixed. If there is gross displacement of the fracture fragments, these should be reduced and a below-knee back-slab applied. The foot should be immediately elevated and ice pack applied. A check X-ray in the back-slab should be taken to confirm reduction. If there is still displacement further reduction is required.

Dislocated/subluxed ankle

Subluxation of the talus in the ankle mortise occurs usually with a displaced bimalleolar/trimalleolar fracture. The position of the ankle should be improved in A&E with reduction and back-slab, and the fracture treated as above. A frank dislocation implies complete loss of contact between the talus and the distal tibia/fibula and needs to be reduced urgently. It is very unlikely to occur in the absence of fracture, due to the level of trauma involved. Again, once the dislocation is reduced, the ankle should be splinted and elevated, and referred for orthopaedic assessment.

FEMORAL SHAFT FRACTURES

Femoral shaft fractures imply high-velocity forces and are rarely isolated injuries. They are potentially life-threatening injuries, with high morbidity and mortality (up to 5%), and need to be dealt with as such. ATLS protocols apply, and all patients should be assessed fully.

Fat embolism is a recognised complication of both the fracture and the treatment, which is intramedullary nailing. Marrow fat can enter the blood stream at the time of injury or during surgery, and travel to the lungs and brain. Symptoms can be subclinical or minor, ranging from mild hypoxia, low-grade pyrexia and tachycardia to florid fat embolisation syndrome – ARDS, central nervous system (CNS) depression, petechial and retinal haemorrhages, jaundice and blood dyscrasia. Florid fat embolism syndrome can be fatal in 5–15% cases. The diagnosis is clinical, and initial management is symptomatic and supportive with adequate fluid and oxygen resuscitation. These patients often need HDU/ITU monitoring, and senior orthopaedic and anaesthetic advice should be sought early if the condition is suspected.

Management

- History – mechanism of injury, road traffic accident, fall, etc.
- ATLS assessment
- Fractures should be clinically detected during secondary survey and should be splinted in a well-padded Thoma splint prior to X-rays. Skin traction should be applied as part of splinting
- Check distal pulses to rule-out femoral artery injury. Examine for open injury. Check distal sensation
- X-rays: lateral C-spine, CXR, pelvis **mandatory**. Full-length femur X-rays in splint including hip and knee
- Large-bore iv × 2.2 litres Hartmann's stat
- FBC, U&E, coagulation, group and save, crossmatch 4 units
- Intravenous analgesia – cyclimorph/morphine titrate to pain
- Keep fasting until **urgent** orthopaedic review

TIBIAL SHAFT FRACTURES

Most tibial shaft fractures are treated surgically – intramedullary nailing or external fixation – to facilitate early rehabilitation for the patient, although some fractures are amenable to conservative treatment.

All patients with tibial shaft fractures should be admitted for elevation and analgesia because of the risk of compartment syndrome, even if the fracture is undisplaced.

The classic scenario is the young male athlete who had sustained a transverse mid-shaft fracture from a direct blow on the football pitch. His already tense, vascular muscle compartment swells and bleeds after the soft-tissue injury, as well as the fracture, and puts him at high risk of compartment syndrome.

Management
- History
- Clinical assessment – distal pulses, distal sensation. Skin for open wounds
- Check for compartment syndrome – pain on passive stretch of toes, muscular tension. The 6 Ps (see page 123) are late signs!
- Above-knee back slab – immobilises ankle and knee and prevents further movement of fracture fragments
- Intravenous line, iv fluids if required
- FBC, U&E, coagulation, group and save
- Intravenous/intramuscular analgesia. Titrate to pain
- Elevate and ice packs
- Regular monitoring for compartment syndrome

HUMERAL SHAFT FRACTURES

Humeral shaft fractures can be high- or low-velocity injuries. There are various treatment options for humeral shaft fractures (including surgical neck/proximal shaft fractures) – they can often be treated non-operatively in functional humeral braces. However, if the fracture is displaced or angulated, the patient should be discussed with the orthopaedic team as treatment decisions depend on the fracture, patient factors – hand dominance, occupation, functional demand, co-morbidities, other injuries – and surgeon preference.

Management

- History
- Clinical assessment – check distal pulses and sensation, particularly the radial nerve
- Distal third shaft fractures have a higher risk of radial nerve palsy as the nerve courses posteriorly around the humerus at this level – (Holstein–Lewis fracture)
- Immobilise in U-slab + sling
- FBC, U&E, coagulation, group + save in case patient is to go to the operation theatre
- Intravenous/intramuscular analgesia. Titrate to pain

FOREARM FRACTURES

The forearm comprises the radius and ulna, which form a pseudo-joint responsible for supination and pronation movements. Displacement of these fractures in either or both bones cannot be accepted, as healing in non-anatomical positions will lead to loss of movement and function.

Remember to always assess the proximal and distal radio-ulnar joints both clinically and radiologically, particularly in single-bone fractures – Monteggia- and Galeazzi-type injuries.

Compartment syndrome can occur in forearm injuries, particularly high-velocity and crush injuries.

Management

- History
- Clinical assessment – distal pulses, sensation and movement
- Tenderness radial head/proximal radio-ulnar joint, and at the distal radio-ulnar joint in the wrist
- Check passive stretch of fingers in extension
- Above-elbow back-slab in elbow flexion + neutral rotation
- Regular monitoring for compartment syndrome
- Intravenous/intramuscular analgesia. Titrate to pain

See Table 5.12.

Table 5.12 Complications of fractures

Immediate	Neurovascular injury Open fractures Haemorrhage
Intraoperative	Neurovascular injury Cardiorespiratory event Reperfusion injury 2° tourniquet usage
Postoperative – early	Wound infection Secondary haemorrhage/anaemia DVT/PE Compartment syndrome Fat embolism ARDS
Postoperative – late	Osteomyelitis Sinus formation Delayed union Non-union Malunion Joint stiffness Loss of range of motion Reflex sympathetic dystrophy Volkmann's ischaemic contracture Heterotropic ossification

There are many causes of knee swelling and a thorough history will usually indicate the diagnosis. Acute trauma causing haemarthrosis will yield a swollen knee and an underlying fracture will need to be ruled out. Rupture of the anterior cruciate ligament (ACL) usually causes immediate swelling, whereas meniscal or ligamentous injuries cause more gradual swelling over 24 hours.

Septic arthritis may occur spontaneously or as a complication of infection elsewhere. The patient will present with a history of acute-onset pain, swelling, loss of movement and increased temperature in the knee. There may be other features of systemic infection such as fever, malaise, nausea, rigors, etc. CRP and ESR are raised in acute infection. This is an important diagnosis to make early, as any delay can lead to complications such as post-infective arthritis, septicaemia and chronic sinus formation.

Reiter's syndrome is a reactive arthritis that occurs usually following chlamydial infection, and is a less common cause of knee swelling. Early recognition and treatment with tetracycline may shorten duration of illness. (*Salmonella*, *Shigella*, *Campylobacter* and *Yersinia* may also be causes of this syndrome). It may affect other large joints, and may involve several joints at once. Only a minority will have the classic triad of symptoms: conjunctivitis, urethritis and arthritis.

Gonorrhoea is the most common form of septic arthritis in young adults and may be associated with more disseminated disease. It is important to take a sexual history in adult patients presenting to A&E with an acute swollen knee, in whom there is no history of trauma. Failure to do so may lead to unrecognised sexually transmitted disease (STD). It is important in all cases to take bloods for FBC, U&E, coagulation, CRP, ESR, cultures, group + save.

See Table 5.13 for assessment of the acute swollen knee.

Table 5.13 Assessment of the acute swollen knee

	History	Exam	X-ray	Management
ACL rupture	Twisting injury. Immediate swelling (tends to be a more severe injury than for a meniscal injury)	Knee effusion ± patellar tap; difficult to assess anterior drawer test acutely	May be avulsion of tibial spine	RICE (Rest, Ice, Compression, Elevation); crutches; early orthopaedic OPD assessment
Meniscal injury	Twisting injury; swelling occurs over 24 hours	Tender joint line; may be effusion	Nil acute; should rule-out fracture	RICE; weight bearing as tolerated; orthopaedic OPD assessment
Ligamentous injury	Valgus/varus strain	Tender on varus/valgus strain (may be widening on strain if ligament rupture)	Nil acute; rule-out fracture	RICE; weight bearing as tolerated; orthopaedic OPD
Tibial plateau	Fall from a height or varus/valgus strain	Knee effusion, bruising; unable to weight bear	Obvious fracture/ impacted fracture or joint depression; look for asymmetry of the joint space	Orthopaedic referral; above-knee back-slab; elevate; CSM (Circulation, sensation, movement) observation

Continued

Table 5.13 *Continued*

Septic arthritis	Current infection; sudden-onset symptoms with no history of trauma	Tender swollen knee. ↑ temperature erythema, painful ROM	Usually normal in acute infection; after 2 weeks may see evidence of periosteal reaction/ sinus formation	Urgent orthopaedic referral and workup for theatre; DO NOT aspirate in A&E – you may introduce infection!
Reiter's syndrome	Large joint arthritis; urethritis – non-purulent discharge; conjunctivitis; pustular skin lesions	Knee effusion ± patellar tap; pain +; look for other features of Reiter's syndrome	Marginal syndesmophytes	Ortho review to rule-out septic arthritis; STD clinic; tetracycline PO; NSAIDs may be helpful
Gonococcal arthritis	Migratory polyarthralgia precedes arthritis in 50%; fever, dermatitis and history of exposure	30–40% of patients with disseminated GC infection present with classic hot, swollen, purulent joint	Nil on acute X-ray; generally less destructive than staphylococcal arthritis	Orthopaedic review; Workup in case of disseminated infection

COMPARTMENT SYNDROME

This is an orthopaedic emergency and early clinical diagnosis is crucial to the outcome. Compartment syndrome is defined as a condition in which the circulation and function of tissues within a closed space are compromised by increased pressure within that space. The commonest cause by far is fracture, but any situation that causes a decrease in compartment size or increase in compartment pressure without a fracture can result in the syndrome. It is most common in fractures involving the upper- and middle-third of the tibia, but also occurs commonly in elbow and forearm injuries. Up to 20% of open tibial fractures develop compartment syndrome. Compartment syndrome is made worse by decreased blood flow into an already under-perfused compartment, and therefore hypotensive trauma patients are at an increased chance of developing this syndrome. Compartment syndrome needs to be identified and managed early to prevent permanent loss of function.

- Muscle functional impairment occurs after 2–4 hours and irreversible functional loss after 4–12 hours
- Nerve functional impairment occurs after 30 minutes and irreversible functional loss after 12–24 hours

Compartment syndrome is treated by decompressing the musculofascial compartments, ie fasciotomy, to allow adequate perfusion.

History

Early presenting symptoms can be varied so you need to be highly aware of the potential for compartment syndrome in dealing with patients with fractures, and to recognise the patients who are at high risk of developing compartment syndrome over the next few hours.

Examination

Established compartment syndrome is very dramatic, but by the time the classic **6 Ps** – pain, pallor, pulselessness, paraesthesia, paralysis and 'perishing with cold' (see page 123) – are evident, you have well and truly missed the boat! So be suspicious, and if in doubt get an urgent orthopaedic review. If you think the patient might be developing compartment syndrome – they probably are. Be aware of the unconscious multiply traumatised patient who cannot complain of pain! Often continuous pressure monitoring in ICU is necessary, or fasciotomy if the injury and clinical picture are likely to result in compartment syndrome.

- Commonest and most reliable symptom is **PAIN** that is out of proportion to the clinical situation
- Pain on passive stretch of the affected muscles is an early and reliable, clinically good sign
- A tense swollen muscle compartment is another common clinical sign
- Hypoaesthesia in the distribution of the nerves traversing the compartment. Sensory symptoms and signs are the first indicators of nerve ischaemia
- A motor deficit is a late finding and is associated with irreversible damage to muscles and nerves
- Distal ischaemia and absent pulses are an indication for arteriography
- Compartment pressure gauges can be inaccurate and misleading, and should be used to confirm the presence of compartment syndrome, rather than to diagnose or exclude it. If you are unsure how to use a pressure monitor, do not use it – wait for orthopaedic assessment

Treatment

- Remove all constricting casts and bandages. Reassess the limb
- If patient is in a full cast – then bivalve with a plaster saw, ie split the cast into two halves with two cuts, and do not forget to cut the wool and stocking beneath the cast for full release
- Patients require urgent decompression (fasciotomy) if symptoms persist
- Treat underlying fracture as per general fracture management
- Keep fasting in case of need for surgery
- **Urgent orthopaedic review**

OTHER CAUSES OF COMPARTMENT SYNDROME

- Severe soft tissue injury
- Crush injuries
- High-pressure injections
- Extravasated blood into tissues
- Gunshot injuries
- Infection
- Iatrogenic – cast too tight
- Reperfusion injuries – following vascular repairs (see Chapter 3)
- Burns – circumferential burns around extremity

INJURIES REQUIRING ORTHOPAEDIC ASSESSMENT

- Spinal injuries
- Open fractures
- Fracture involving a joint with displacement
- Fracture with neurovascular compromise
- Fractures with angulation/displacement or rotation
- Fracture dislocations
- Hip fractures
- Femoral shaft fractures
- Tibial shaft fractures
- Forearm fractures
- Septic arthritis
- Compartment syndrome

CHAPTER 6

CARDIOTHORACIC SURGERY

M O MURPHY AND K E McLAUGHLIN

INTRODUCTION

Thoracic surgery represents a great deal of the 'on-call' workload of cardiothoracic surgery, dealing with regional and local referrals for malignant, inflammatory, infective or traumatic disease of the chest and lungs. Many of the difficulties associated with thoracic surgery surround the mysteries of chest drains and the significance of words such as 'swing', 'suction' and 'leak'. Chest drain management is a controversial area of medicine with many inconsistencies between surgeons and sometimes within surgeons! The common pathologies are discussed with particular attention to the mysteries of the drain.

Cardiac surgery is generally limited to specialist units often separate from the main hospital. There is likely to be a resident surgeon looking after postoperative patients on the ITU. There is little in the way of hospital referrals to cardiac surgical services apart from acute cardiology cases, which are often consultant to consultant. Because of this the majority of cardiac surgical workload is surgical or intensive care based.

LUNG CANCER

Carcinoma of the lung remains an extremely important cause of death in the UK. The disease has a strong association with smoking and exposure to occupational or environmental carcinogens. The prognosis of patients with lung cancer has changed very little over the years despite various developments. Tumours are described by histological subtypes but from a management point of view should be regarded as either small-cell or non-small-cell carcinoma. Although surgery offers the best chance of cure, the majority of lung cancer is inoperable at the time of diagnosis. In this setting patient life can be extended through the use of chemotherapy and radiotherapy. Surgery is also used to palliate end-stage disease by drainage of pleural effusions or endo-bronchial therapy for obstruction.

History

Patients may present either with clinical signs and symptoms (below) or an incidental finding on CXR or CT scan performed for another reason (such as before CABG). Classic clinical presentation with lung cancer is related to the tumour itself or loco-regional spread or the systemic manifestations of disseminated disease. These include:

- Cough
- Haemoptysis
- Shortness of breath
- Pneumonia
- Weight loss
- Lethargy
- Change in voice
- Pain
- Dysphagia

Examination

Patients may be breathless and have co-existent obstructive, restrictive or fibrotic parenchymal lung disease. It is important to assess for the presence of effusions and lymphadenopathy. Many patients have evidence of weight loss and clubbing. Locally or systemically disseminated disease may be indicated by:

- Malignant pleural effusion
- Scalene lymphadenopathy (posterior triangle)
- Hepatic invasion
- Superior vena cava obstruction
- Horner's syndrome

Investigations

In many patients the cancer is discovered through routine CXR, but this is a limited tool to stage disease. Staging can be achieved by a combination of CT scanning and bronchoscopy, both of which can facilitate fine needle aspiration biopsy. Patients are often referred to a thoracic surgeon for investigations to aid diagnosis – open biopsy, rigid bronchoscopy and biopsy or mediastinoscopy for nodal biopsy. Occasionally, cytological examination of the sputum may also yield a tissue diagnosis.

It is essential to assess those patients considered suitable for resection with pulmonary function tests to see if they would tolerate a curative resection. Increasingly positron emission tomography (PET) is replacing mediastinoscopy to distinguish patients with resectable disease from patients who are better served by radiotherapy/chemotherapy. It is worthwhile carrying out preoperative ABG in patients considered for resection as those with raised carbon dioxide do poorly, and the preoperative pO_2 will provide a realistic goal of oxygen saturation postoperatively.

Treatment

Surgical resection of the tumour offers the best prospect of survival. Operative mortality has consistently been close to 5% with a third of survivors making it to 5 years. Chemo- and radiotherapy also have a major role either alone or in association with surgery. Thoracic surgeons are equally involved in the palliation of lung cancer through talc pleurodesis for pleural effusion and endobronchial therapy for airway obstruction.

In patients with suitable respiratory function and curable disease on staging with CT scan/PET scan/mediastinoscopy/biopsy, wedge, lobe or lung resection offer long-term cure. Small-cell carcinomas are less likely to be amenable to surgery than non-small-cell, with only a small percentage of patients suitable for resection at presentation. Patients with locally advanced disease are treated with chemotherapy.

EMPYEMA

This is an intrapleural collection of pus most commonly as a consequence of pneumonia. Empyema may also complicate lung abscesses, thoracic surgery or chest drain insertion.

History

Patients often present with swinging fevers and pyrexia following an episode of pneumonia, thoracic surgery or chest drain insertion. When large, an empyema may also manifest as breathlessness.

Examination

Patients can look generally unwell with classical clinical features of dullness and decreased air entry with finger clubbing.

Investigations

- CXR may reveal basal effusion and pleural aspiration will show pus cells in the fluid
- CT scan will further delineate the anatomy of the cavity and the presence of loculation as well as any underlying lung disease

Treatment

Early adequate chest drainage may facilitate resolution of the empyema. Large, loculated or prolonged episodes often necessitate removal of the focus at surgery, performed as a video-assisted thoracic surgery (VATS) procedure or through open decortication. Culture and sensitivity of the cavity aspirates should guide antibiotic therapy. Failure of adequate drainage with or without decortication should raise the possibility of an underlying condition preventing adequate healing. For example:

- Broncho-pleural fistula
- Tuberculosis
- Carcinoma
- Bronchiectasis
- Foreign body
- Subphrenic abscess

PNEUMOTHORAX

Air in the pleural space, from whatever cause, is called a pneumothorax. It is described according to the cause:

- **Spontaneous** – in the absence of external instrumentation or trauma
- **Traumatic** – following injury with or without rib fracture
- **Iatrogenic** – following central line insertion, pleural aspiration or chest drain removal

Another classification is based on the source of air, which is either open in the case of surgery, aspiration, central line or trauma, or closed in the case of leakage of air from lung tissue or oesophagus. In closed pneumothoraces, tension pneumothorax may occur due to the build-up of pressure in the pleural cavity with mediastinal shift and compression of the contralateral lung.

Spontaneous pneumothorax tends to occur in two groups: young patients with apical blebs (tall thin men) and older patients, caused by rupture of emphysematous bullae. Iatrogenic pneumothoraces are frequently picked up on post-procedural CXR. Traumatic pneumothorax may be associated with relatively trivial trauma with isolated pneumothorax, or as part of a polytrauma with haemopneumothorax with lung injury and possible tension.

History

Should concentrate on:

- Any previous episodes
- Pulmonary disease
- Recent history of trauma or procedure

Examination

Patients present with dyspnoea and decreased air entry over a hyper-resonant lung. Patients should always be assessed for tracheal shift and cardiovascular compromise of tension pneumothorax prior to CXR.

Investigations

CXR is often adequate to make decisions on treatment but future investigation with CT scan is warranted in complicated cases where underlying lung parenchymal disease may exist. Tension pneumothorax should be a clinical diagnosis.

Treatment

In most cases intercostal drainage will be required as described below. Small pneumothoraces can be treated conservatively with regular CXR to confirm resorption of air by the pleura or by needle aspiration. When there is loculation or adherence in parts to the chest wall it may be safer to treat conservatively or carry out a VATS procedure as these cases have high complication rates.

When there is a suspicion of tension it is essential to treat prior to CXR with initial decompression through the second intercostal space in the mid-clavicular line with a large vascular cannula followed by formal chest drain insertion on the affected side. Drainage for 48 hours is often sufficient to allow for lung expansion without air leak and the drain can be confidently removed.

In cases of recurrent pneumothorax, prolonged air leak or a suspicion of previous contralateral pneumothorax, surgical pleurodesis or pleurectomy is indicated. This procedure involves the creation of irritated parietal and visceral pleura, which will then adhere to each other during adequate re-expansion using chest drains. This can be achieved by mechanical abrasion of the pleura or the use of talc. In pleurectomy, the parietal pleura is removed and the visceral pleura adheres to the chest wall, obliterating the pleural space.

PLEURAL EFFUSION

Pleural effusion is described as either an exudate (high protein content) or transudate (low protein content) of fluid in the pleural space.

CAUSES OF TRANSUDATE EFFUSIONS

- Cardiac, renal and hepatic failure
- Hypothyroidism
- Meige's syndrome.

CAUSES OF AN EXUDATE

- Malignancy
- Pneumonia
- Tuberculosis
- Pancreatitis
- Ovarian cancer
- Various connective tissue diseases

History

It is often associated with progressive breathlessness, depending on underlying pathology. It is important to elicit any past history suggestive of chronic cardiac, hepatic or renal insufficiency, chest infections, tuberculosis, connective tissue disease or malignancy.

Examination

The classic signs of decreased breath sounds over an area of stony, dull sound on percussion can be accompanied by bronchial breathing above the fluid level.

Investigations

CXR will confirm diagnosis with characteristic meniscus. Pleural fluid should be sent for microbiological examination including for tuberculosis, biochemistry for LDH and amylase and cytological examination for malignant cells. Final diagnosis may require pleural or bronchoscopic biopsy for transudates.

Treatment

In general, treatment of the underlying cause will result in resolution of the effusion while the presence of blood, air or an exudate may necessitate drainage for either diagnostic and therapeutic reasons. Thoracoscopy allows tissue diagnosis and drainage of the pleura space and facilitates pleurodesis.

POSTOPERATIVE CARE OF THORACIC PATIENTS

The postoperative management of thoracic surgery patients has much in common with that of postoperative general surgical patients with a heavy emphasis on pain relief, adequate ventilation and fluid balance.

VATS patients generally have had a minor surgical insult and once pain free most of their care surrounds the function and removal of their drains. In many VATS procedures apical (air) and basal (fluid) drains are sited, but there is much variation among surgeons with regard to the place for suction and the order and timing of drain removal. In the presence of adequately positioned and functioning drains and a postoperative pneumothorax most will advocate the use of suction in an attempt to remove air from the cavity and facilitate attachment of the lung to the chest wall. If the basal or fluid drain is draining little it is worth removing. The absence of a swing in the level of the underwater seal implies the lung is well expanded or the drain is in the wrong place. A well-expanded lung, and an apical drain with no 'air leak' and minimal swing usually warrants drain removal.

In addition to the above drain-related issues, lung-resection patients require close monitoring of hydration status. Patients who have had lobectomy or pneumonectomy are prone to acute lung injury with dire consequences. The combination of a large surgical insult, fluid sequestration and loss of vasomotor tone with epidurals renders these patients at high risk of hypotension and oliguria. However, it is essential not to over-hydrate these patients as ARDS secondary to pulmonary oedema, particular following pneumonectomy, has an extremely high mortality. While it is obviously important to replace losses and prescribe adequate maintenance fluid this should be done carefully. It is common to maintain blood pressure with the vasoconstrictor, noradrenaline, to counteract the vasodilatation of the epidural and allow a low hourly infusion volume (sometimes accepting relative oligura).

As with any thoracic intervention it is essential to carry out a postoperative CXR to monitor events within the pleura. Patients should be counselled on the importance of deep breathing and expectorating. Blood gas analysis will guide oxygen therapy and the need to decrease or increase the fraction of inspired oxygen (FiO_2). Preoperative ABG analysis will provide a realistic target for pO_2.

Chest drain management in pneumonectomy patients can seem unusual as the priority is to fill rather than drain the operated side to prevent mediastinal shift. At pneumonectomy, the entire lung on the side of the lesion is removed, creating a large potential space. Some surgeons place a drain in the chest which allows assessment and management of post operative blood loss. The tube is then clamped with short periods of unclamping thereafter to adjust the pressure. It is important to leave the drain clamped because if the patient coughs, a large amount of air can be displaced with mediastinal shift to the operated side. In this situation air or fluid needs to be re-admitted to correct the displacement.

Immediately postoperatively the operated cavity contains air. During the next 24–36 hours the fluid level rises as carbon dioxide is absorbed and air is expelled through the wound with resulting subcutaneous emphysema. This fluid, composed of retained blood and inflammatory exudate, consistently rises with further absorption of the intra-thoracic air. The volume of the fluid-filled cavity may be adjusted to maintain a central position of the mediastinum. Over the subsequent months the cavity becomes completely fluid filled, resulting in the classic opaque hemithorax following pneumonectomy.

One of the most serious complications of pneumonectomy is broncho-pleural fistula and is usually heralded by 'rusty' or blood-stained sputum. The connection between the tracheal air and pleura allows a change from decreased breath sounds to clear vocal resonance and is reason enough to warrant daily auscultation of patients following pneumonectomy. In addition, the CXR shows changes, with widening of the apical air space, tracheal shift away from the operated side (rather than towards the operated side) and resorption of fluid to the extent that eventually the entire space is taken over by air. Treatment of large or significant fistula is by pleural drainage and elective repair.

BLEEDING

While the sudden haemorrhage of slipped tie of a major vessel is often fatal, the slow bleeding from a bronchial or intercostal vessel gradually fills the chest with blood. Unlike lobectomy patients, where such bleeding is obvious from increased drainage, pneumonectomy patients need to be carefully monitored for occult bleeding. Excessive drainage of serous fluid post-pneumonectomy should raise the suspicion of infection

---

CHEST DRAINS

DO'S AND DON'TS

The differential diagnosis between a pneumothorax and bullous disease requires careful radiological assessment. Similarly it is important to differentiate between the presence of collapse and a pleural effusion when the chest radiograph shows a unilateral 'whiteout'. Lung densely adherent to the chest wall throughout the hemithorax is an absolute contraindication to chest drain insertion. During the insertion of a chest tube in a patient on a high pressure ventilator (especially with positive end-expiratory pressure (PEEP)), it is essential to disconnect from the ventilator at the time of insertion to avoid injury.

Vasovagal reactions and death due to vagal stimulation following tube insertion support the use of analgesia or sedative unless there are contraindications to their use. Both these classes of drugs may cause respiratory depression and patients with underlying lung disease such as chronic obstructive pulmonary disease should be observed, as reversal agents are occasionally necessary. Never put a chest drain in without obsessive checking of patient identification, CXR findings, the side and site needing drainage, and that the clinical findings, CXR and patient all agree that a drain is necessary.

PREPARATION

The preferred position for drain insertion is on a bed, slightly rotated, with the arm on the side of the lesion behind the patient's head to expose the axillary area. Insertion should be in the 'safe triangle' bordered by the anterior border of the latissimus dorsi, the lateral border of the pectoralis major muscle, a line superior to the horizontal level of the nipple, and an apex below the axilla. This position minimises risk to underlying structures such as the internal mammary artery and avoids damage to muscle and breast tissue resulting in unsightly scarring.

A chest tube should not be inserted without further image guidance if free air or fluid cannot be aspirated with a needle prior to insertion. Imaging should be used to select the appropriate site for chest tube placement and a chest radiograph must be available at the time of drain insertion except in the case of tension pneumothorax. Aseptic technique is essential to avoid wound site infection or secondary empyema.

The use of prophylactic antibiotics to cover chest drain insertion is controversial but is probably indicated in trauma.

INSERTION

Local anaesthetic is infiltrated to raise a dermal bleb before deeper infiltration of the intercostal muscles and pleural surface. Low concentration should be used because the volume given is considered to be more important than the dose, to aid spread of the effective anaesthetic area.

Ensure that sufficient time has elapsed before starting. Once the anaesthetic has taken effect an incision is made. This should be slightly bigger than the operator's finger and tube. The incision should be made just above and parallel to a rib to take into account the elevation of tissue with raising of the arm. Blunt dissection of the subcutaneous tissue and muscle into the pleural cavity has become universal.

A path is made through the chest wall – using a Spencer–Wells clamp or similar – by opening the clamp to separate the muscle fibres. This track should be explored with a finger through into the thoracic cavity to ensure there are no underlying organs that might be damaged at tube insertion and that there are no pleural adhesions. The creation of a patent track into the pleural cavity ensures that excessive force is not needed during drain insertion. The position of the tip of the chest tube should ideally be aimed apically for a pneumothorax or basally for fluid. However, any tube position can be effective at draining air or fluid and an effectively functioning drain should not be repositioned solely because of its radiographic position.

Two sutures are usually inserted, the first to assist later closure of the wound after drain removal and the second, a stay suture, to secure the drain. The wound closure suture should be inserted before blunt dissection. A '1 silk mattress' suture across the incision is usually employed. Large amounts of tape and padding to dress the site are unnecessary. A transparent dressing allows the wound site to be inspected by nursing staff for leakage or infection.

CLAMPING DRAIN

A bubbling chest tube should never be clamped. Clamping a chest drain in the presence of a continuing air leak may lead to the potentially fatal complication of tension pneumothorax. Drainage of a large pleural effusion should be controlled to prevent the potential complication of re-expansion pulmonary oedema.

In cases of pneumothorax, clamping of the chest tube should usually be avoided. If a chest tube for pneumothorax is clamped, this should be under the supervision of a respiratory physician or thoracic surgeon, the patient should be managed in a specialist ward with experienced nursing staff, and the patient should not leave the ward environment.

DRAINAGE SYSTEM

All chest tubes should be connected to a single flow drainage system, eg underwater seal bottle or Heimlich's flutter valve. The chest tube is then attached to a drainage system which only allows one direction of flow. This is usually the closed underwater seal bottle in which a tube is placed under water at a depth of approximately 3 cm with a side vent in the drain which allows escape of air, or connection to a suction pump. This enables the operator to see the air bubble come out as the lung re-expands in the case of pneumothorax or fluid evacuation rate in empyemas, pleural effusions, or haemothorax. The continuation of bubbling suggests a continued visceral pleural air leak, although it may also occur in patients on suction when the drain is partly out of the thorax and one of the tube holes is open to the air.

The respiratory swing in the fluid in the chest tube is useful for assessing tube patency and confirms the position of the tube in the pleural cavity. The disadvantages of the underwater seal system include obligatory inpatient management, difficulty of patient mobilisation, and the risk of knocking over the bottle. Use of a flutter valve system allows earlier mobilisation and the potential for earlier discharge of patients with chest drains. Flutter valves cannot be used with fluid drainage as they tend to become blocked.

SUCTION

When chest drain suction is required, a high-volume/low-pressure system should be used. A high-volume pump (eg Vernon–Thompson) is required to cope with a large leak. A low-volume pump (eg Roberts pump) is inappropriate as it is unable to cope with the rapid flow, thereby effecting a situation similar to clamping and risking formation of a tension pneumothorax. A wall suction adaptor may also be effective, although chest drains must not be connected directly to the high negative pressure available from wall suction.

POSTINSERTION CARE

A CXR should be taken after insertion of a chest drain to assess tube position, exclude complications such as pneumothorax or surgical emphysema, and assess the success of the procedure in the volume of fluid drainage or pneumothorax resolution. If an underwater seal is used, instructions must be given to keep the bottle below the insertion site at all times, to keep it upright, and to ensure that adequate water is in the system to cover the end of the tube.

Daily assessment of the amount of drainage/bubbling and the presence of respiratory swing should be documented, preferably on a dedicated chest drain chart. Instruction with regard to chest drain clamping, these must be clearly recorded.

REMOVAL OF THE CHEST TUBE

The chest tube should be removed either while the patient performs Valsalva's manoeuvre or during expiration with a brisk firm movement while an assistant ties the previously placed closure suture. The timing of removal depends on the original reason for insertion and clinical progress

In the case of pneumothorax, the drain should not usually be removed until bubbling has ceased and a CXR demonstrates lung re-inflation.

PREOPERATIVE CARE OF CARDIAC PATIENTS

There are many distinctions between preoperative assessment of cardiac patients and other surgical patients and so this is discussed separately in this chapter (in addition to the preoperative assessment describe in Chapter 1, pages 10–18).

PULSE OXIMETER

This is an essential preoperative test and if less than 95% on air then investigate appropriately with ABG and/or pulmonary function tests. This is as much for preoperative detection and optimisation of impaired respiratory function as to set realistic targets during the postoperative recovery.

COAGULATION PROFILE

This is needed for patients on anticoagulants and with a history of bleeding diathesis.

LIVER FUNCTION TESTS

Liver function tests should be performed for patients with a history of alcohol consumption in excess of recommendations (28 units for men, 21 units for women), jaundice, viral hepatitis, hepatotoxic drugs, signs of hepatomegaly, lymphadenopathy, jaundice and right heart failure.

X-RAYS

A CXR within 3/12 is acceptable unless there has been a change in clinical symptoms that would warrant an X-ray. Patients with rheumatoid arthritis and cervical spondylosis should have a cervical spine X-ray. All re-do cardiac surgical patients should have a lateral CXR or a CT scan to assess the location of mediastinal structures in relation to the sternum.

CAROTID DOPPLER

There is conflicting evidence for combined carotid endarterectomy and CABG and so the indication for **carotid Doppler** is controversial and warrants discussion with the operating surgeon.

ECG

ECG performed less than a month ago is generally adequate unless there have been new symptoms.

SMOKERS

Smokers have increased postoperative morbidity (chest infection, respiratory failure, prolonged ITU and hospital stay) and long-term reduction in the benefits of surgery (accelerated graft failure after bypass surgery) and so should be extensively counselled prior to surgery. For maximum benefit patients need to have stopped smoking 2–4 weeks preoperatively, but it is worth noting that carboxyhaemoglobin levels fall to normal in approximately 24 hours while mucociliary function and bronchial secretion production may take up to 4 weeks to return to normal.

MEDICATION

Angiotensin-converting enzyme (ACE) inhibitors, angiotensin-II receptor antagonists and β-blockers should continue until the day before surgery. The anaesthetist will usually specify in their pre-med instructions what drugs are to be given on the day of surgery. Aspirin dose should be reduced to 75 mg until surgery. For many operations it is important to stop antiplatelet therapy in stable/elective patients a few days before surgery unless the clinical scenario indicates otherwise eg acute coronary syndrome.

ISCHAEMIC HEART DISEASE

History

it is essential to look for any risk factors for coronary disease such as smoking, diabetes, hypertension, hypercholesterolaemia, dietary, family history. It is also important to identify co-morbidities which may affect the outcome of surgery such as renal impairment, diabetes, coexistent peripheral vascular disease or history of cerebrovascular disease.

Examination

Assess for stigmata of smoking, hypercholesterolaemia, peripheral vascular disease, varicose veins, previous cardiac or thoracic surgery, murmurs and evidence of restrictive, obstructive or fibrotic lung disease. Allan's test of radial artery function is carried out particularly in patients with limited available conduits such as those requiring redo-CABG or patients with varicose veins.

Investigations

Because of common risk factors of smoking and age, it is always important to assess for any lung masses on CXR. All patients will have been referred via a cardiologist so are likely to have already been investigated with ECG, routine bloods such as FBC, fasting glucose, cholesterol and coronary angiography.

Treatment

Medical therapy

Medical therapy for coronary artery disease has improved greatly over the years through a succession of randomised control trials to characterise the optimal management in terms of symptomatic relief and survival. Foremost among these have been the widespread use of antiplatelet agents such as aspirin and most recently clopidogrel. On the basis of the success of these agents in chronic ischaemic heart disease, antithrombotics of various classes are now used in acute coronary syndrome (ACS). MI is usually described as either acute MI with the traditional ECG changes or a non-ST elevation MI. The latter is part of the acute coronary syndrome, where there is biochemical evidence of myocardial damage without the classic ECG findings. Agents used in the treatment of ACS include antiplatelet agents, thrombolytics, GP II–IIIb inhibitors and heparin.

Symptomatic improvement in patients with coronary disease occurs with use of anti-anginals such as nitrates, nicorandil and β-blockers. Prognostic benefit in terms of survival and decreased cardiovascular events is seen with ACE inhibitors, β-blockers and statins. There is also strong evidence for improved survival with risk factor modification such as smoking cessation, BP control (regardless of agent), diabetic control, weight reduction, dietary modification and exercise.

Interventional therapy

In addition to this extensive array of therapies, interventional therapy has evolved. This includes percutaneous coronary intervention (PCI) and coronary artery bypass grafting (CABG) for both acute and chronic disease. Central to both treatment modalities is the treatment of stenotic atherosclerotic coronary lesions on angiography to improve the patient's symptoms and/or prognosis. Lesions on angiography which demonstrate a reduction in luminal diameter of 50% indicate a 75% reduction in luminal narrowing and are described as significant. Disease is classified by artery and distribution and usually is described as either affecting or sparing the left main stem and how many of the three main coronaries are significantly narrowed. PCI uses various techniques but most commonly this involves balloon angioplasty with or without the use of a metal stent which may be drug-eluting. Surgery involves using autologous conduits such as the internal mammary arteries (IMA) and the long saphenous vein to bypass the culprit lesions.

Surgery is preferred over PCI in those patients with left main stem disease and three vessel coronary disease. Urgent surgery is carried out on those in whom PCI has been unsuccessful or on those who have the above disease pattern with crescendo symptoms. It is worth noting that those who have had a non-ST elevation MI are at extremely high risk of having an MI in the subsequent 6 months without intervention.

VALVULAR DISEASE

Cardiac valves may be affected by a variety of pathological processes. These include rheumatic heart disease, infection, degeneration, and functional pathology (fibrous ring dilation). There can be associated conditions, such as connective tissue disease and collagen vascular diseases. Although many medications are available for the palliation of valvular disease, definitive treatment requires surgery.

Valve dysfunction can manifest in a number of ways. Whether the pathology is valve stenosis or regurgitation, ultimately symptoms of heart failure will develop. Infection occurs where blood-borne pathogens colonise the valve causing a combination of sepsis, valve destruction and embolisation. In general valves with pre-existing disease or abnormalities, such as previous rheumatic fever, valve surgery or congenital abnormalities, are more susceptible to infection/abscess formation than normal valves. This tends to affect the left-sided valves, with right-sided infective lesions predominantly affecting intravenous drug misusers and patients with endocardial permanent pacemakers.

Various subtleties of pathology and indications for intervention exist among this heterogeneous patient group but in general when the risks and prognosis of the valvular defect outweigh the risk of surgery, the patient should be considered for valve replacement/repair. This is most commonly carried out using cardiopulmonary bypass and diastolic arrest (cardioplegia) to allow for the safe opening of the cardiac chambers. The valve in question is inspected for suitability for repair or the necessity of replacement. In general the aortic and pulmonary valve is resected and replaced whereas the mitral and tricuspid valves are increasingly repaired or reinforced (metal ring) rather than replaced. In most cases either a mechanical or a tissue (bovine pericardial or porcine) valve is implanted. Mechanical valves are extremely durable but require lifelong warfarin therapy for prevention of thromboembolic events. Tissue valves are less durable than mechanical valves but do not require lifelong warfarin and patients are usually prescribed aspirin for prevention of thromboembolic events. Alternative valve substitutes include homografts which are particularly useful in the setting of acute endocarditis and the Ross procedure (pulmonary autograft).

In the setting of endocarditis the patient is often treated as a matter of urgency and it is important to administer appropriate high dose intravenous antibiotics. Surgery involves extensive removal of any infected tissue at surgery prior to valve repair/replacement. As tissue valves are more resistant to infection, surgeons tend to place these valves in the setting of endocarditis.

AORTIC DISEASE

Thoracic aortic disease may involve the aortic root as it emerges from the left ventricle, the ascending aorta, aortic arch or descending aorta.

Aortic aneurysm may be complicated by acute dissection or rupture with extremely high mortality. Surgery is indicated to prevent these complications and is usually considered when the aneurysm reaches a particular size. In patients with Marfan's Syndrome regular follow up is undertaken to assess the aortic root dimensions and surgery is undertaken early in the process to prevent rupture or dissection.

The operative techniques are complex and these procedures are associated with a significant risk of morbidity and mortality. Aortic root surgery may require aortic valve replacement, surgery involving the arch may utilise deep hypothermic circulatory arrest for cerebral protection and procedures on the descending aorta are associated with a significant risk of spinal cord ischaemia and paraplegia.

An increasing number of patients with aneurysm of the descending thoracic aorta are managed with endovascular stent graft technology.

Acute aortic dissection involving the ascending aorta is a surgical emergency and requires urgent surgery to prevent death from rupture or malperfusion. When acute aortic dissection is confined to the descending aorta, initial management is medical. Surgery may be required if there is rupture, malperfusion or failure of medical therapy. Interventional radiology has an increasingly valuable role to play in this setting.

PACING WIRES

Placement of epicardial pacing wires allows external pacing of the heart. They may be used intraoperatively to facilitate weaning the patient from cardiopulmonary bypass or in the postoperative period when rhythm problems such as heart block and bradycardia may require treatment. By convention epicardial pacing wires exiting on the left side of the chest are ventricular while those on the right are atrial. Often patients will only have ventricular wires. Active wires are embedded in the myocardium while for indifferent or inactive wires, the end is in the chest wall. If there is only a single wire then it will be an active ventricular wire on the left side of the chest. To pace successfully an indifferent wire will need to be placed in the skin:

- Get a pacing wire
- Push the needle through the skin somewhere near the other pacing wire
- Ensure that the bare section of wire is in the skin
- Break off the needle and connect to the pacing box
- Finally, secure the wire so that it does not pull out
- Connect the pacing wires to the pacing lead and the lead to the pacing box

If all of the wires are active it does not really matter how they are connected. If there is an active and an indifferent wire the active wire will usually be the shorter of the two. When connecting the leads the convention is that **black is ACTIVE**. Connect the ventricular leads to the ventricular terminals of the box and the atrial leads to the atrial terminals. Set the pacing box to DDD 500 (see below). This limits the ventricular rate when sequentially pacing in case the patient goes into fast atrial fibrillation. Set the rate to 70–90 beats per minute and increase threshold until capture occurs. Whenever possible pace atrially or sequentially (ie atrial and ventricular pacing). Adjust rate to achieve optimum blood pressure. Careful note should be made of the pacing threshold. This will require careful attention if pacing is required for more than a few days. Do not disconnect the pacing box to observe the underlying rhythm. On the first postoperative morning it is necessary to identify the underlying rhythm in those who have been paced over night. Slowly turn down the ventricular rate and observe the pacing threshold and spontaneous rate. If possible obtain an ECG with the pacemaker off to categorise the degree and type of block. If pacing is still required after 5 days a permanent pacemaker may be needed

EPICARDIAL PACING

Pacing can be fixed, demand or sequential. Fixed pacing paces the heart at a predetermined rate and ignores the patient's underlying rate whereas demand pacing only triggers when the rate falls below the set rate. Demand pacing is more usefully regarded as background pacing that is inhibited when the patient's heart is beating above a certain rate. When there are atrial and ventricular pacing leads the heart can be sequentially paced by inhibition (demand) or at a set rate (fixed). Electrical activity is sensed in both chambers and pacing occurs either at a fixed or demand protocol to the atria followed after a programmed time to the ventricles.

A THREE-LETTER CODE OF PACEMAKERS

- The first letter – refers to the paced chamber which can be atrium (A), ventricle (V), both or dual (D) or non-paced (O)
- The second letter – likewise refers to the chamber sensed and is described as A, V, D or O
- The third letter – refers to the response of the pacemaker to inhibit (I), trigger (T), both inhibit and trigger (D), or there is no response (O)

Therefore, if you simply wanted to pace the atria regardless of the heart activity you would use AOO, while if you wanted the atria to be paced if the heart rate fell below a certain rate you would set the pacemaker stimulus to be inhibited by atrial contraction but to stimulate the atria below that rate – AAI. Similarly, for the ventricles you would use VOO and VVI. To achieve a sequential pacing the box is set to sense ventricular pacing and then be stimulated to pace the atria and ventricles in a sequential manner – DVI. The most frequently used post operative pacing setting is DDD

POSTOPERATIVE MEDICATION

Postoperative cardiac surgical patients benefit from a variety of medications and this is an ideal opportunity to establish secondary prevention. In particular antiplatelets and statins are an essential consideration for anyone with coronary disease.

Postoperative CABG patients benefit from aspirin particularly at the higher dose of 300 mg for the first year, as this appears to inhibit the proliferative endothelial problem in the veins. If a patient is intolerant of aspirin then most surgeons prescribe clopidogrel 75 mg.

Patients should be on 40 mg of one of the three main statins. Atorvastatin is stronger than simvastatin, which is stronger than pravastatin. In addition atorvastatin is better at lowering triglycerides than the other agents and for these reasons is the preferred therapy. It is important to realise that statins have beneficial effects on blood vessels quite independent of their cholesterol effect.

Several studies have shown that ACE inhibitors prolong life and that this is likely to be a class effect. It is therefore recommended to start (or restart) patients on an ACE inhibitor postoperatively either while as an inpatient or advise their GP. It is important to realise that many hypertensive patients are normotensive postoperatively and that there are high levels of renal artery stenosis in cardiac patients. This means it is essential to monitor renal function in these patients and aim to achieve an appropriate therapeutic dose. There is good evidence supporting Ramipril in patients with ischemic heart disease and it is desirable for most patients to leave the hospital on at least the lower dosage of 2.5 mg. However, if the patient was on an alternative ACE inhibitor or an angiotensin-II receptor antagonist (because of an ACE cough) then that agent should be started again and, in the same way, tiltrated up to the therapeutic dose.

The evidence for taking β-blockers after CABG·is weak but there is evidence that strongly favours β-blockade following an MI. Therefore patients with a history of MI should be started on a β-blocker.

As with most major surgery, patients are at high risk of PE and DVT and so are given thromboprophylaxis with LMWH. This can be stopped when fully mobile and it is important to omit the dose for at least 12 hours after thoracic epidural insertion or removal. TED stockings on both legs may provide addition thromboprophylaxis but early mobilisation should be encouraged. Patients who develop postoperative DVT should receive warfarin (INR 2.0–3.0) for 3 months whereas patients who develop postoperative PE should receive warfarin (INR 2.0–3.0) for 6 months.

Gastrointestinal protection

It is worth prescribing an antacid for gastric mucosal protection against stress ulceration in the early postoperative period but this can be stopped after 2–3 days when the patient is eating. Medications used include ranitidine, sucralfate or a proton pump inhibitor (PPI). It is important to note that a PPI prescribed for suspected GI bleeds works very poorly in the presence of sucralfate, so this should be stopped when commencing a PPI.

Corticosteroids

Patients who have received prolonged therapy with corticosteroids develop adrenal insufficiency which may be persistent. Abrupt withdrawal of corticosteroids may precipitate acute adrenal insufficiency with profound hypotension. It is common to prescribe IV hydrocortisone with the pre-medication prior to surgery and to continue until normal steroid therapy can be reintroduced. It is also essential to appreciate that if the patient is unwell then the hydrocortisone dose may need to be increased.

Non-steroidal anti-inflammatory drugs

These should be prescribed cautiously, particularly in the elderly, due to the high postoperative risk of adverse effects. These include serious gastro-intestinal toxicity such as haemorrhage. There is also risk of renal impairment and bronchospasm. When these are used additional gastric mucosal protection should be considered and the prescription should be limited to 2 days with clinical review prior to re-prescribing.

BLOOD TRANSFUSION

The myocardium is the tissue most at risk of ischaemia secondary to anaemia because myocardial oxygen delivery is flow dependent. Oxygen extraction is near maximal even under normal conditions. Coronary artery disease and ventricular hypertrophy both limit flow thus myocardial oxygen delivery is primarily limited by the oxygen-carrying capacity of the blood. This is determined by the haemoglobin concentration in the blood.

Blood transfusions may be associated with adverse consequences and are expensive. Postoperative anaemia is relatively common and there is no excess mortality in otherwise fit surgical patients with haemoglobin levels down to about 70 g/l (7 g/dl). For young fit patients transfusion is usually only necessary if the anaemia is symptomatic. For older cardiac patients it is preferable to keep the Hb above 80 g/l (8 g/dl) or even 100 g/l (10 g/dl) in some cases such as patients experiencing a complicated recovery with ongoing low cardiac output, multiorgan failure or continuing sepsis. In asymptomatic patients at low risk with haemoglobin 80 g/l (8 g/dl), ferrous sulphate (200 mg three times a day) is an adequate treatment and should increase the haemoglobin by approximately 10 g/l (1 g/dl) per week. One unit of packed cells should increase the haemoglobin by approximately 15 g/l (1.5 g/dl).

A sudden fall in postoperative haemoglobin should arouse suspicion of gastrointestinal bleeding, usually from peptic ulceration in the duodenum or stomach. In this case it is essential to treat with a PPI and have a low threshold for upper gastrointestinal endoscopy.

POTASSIUM AND MAGNESIUM

Patients having cardiopulmonary bypass will need postoperative diuretics to counter the obligatory fluid and electrolyte retention. Patients on diuretics preoperatively may require a higher dose. It is important not to give amiloride in conjunction with ACE inhibitors, angiotensin-II receptor antagonists or spironolactone (all have potassium-sparing effects) due to the risk of hyperkalaemia. Diuretics can be discontinued or the dose reduced when the postoperative daily weight is down to the preoperative level. Patients on preoperative diuretics will usually require long-term postoperative diuretic therapy.

To reduce the risk of postoperative supraventricular tachyarrhythmia serum K^+ should be kept between 4.5 mmol/l and 5.0 mmol/l. The routine use of the potassium-sparing diuretics in addition to loop diuretics can decrease the often significant use of oral and iv supplementation. Hypomagnesaemia results from diuretic therapy. It can result in arrhythmias and may result in a secondary hypokalaemia. This hypokalaemia is resistant to K^+ supplements until the hypomagnesaemia has also been corrected. Magnesium loading should be carried out postoperatively prior to potassium correction, as the main problem is a combination of low magnesium with low potassium. It is important to only prescribe potassium supplements for 48 hours and check serum levels every other day or more frequently if clinically indicated.

For supraventricular arrhythmias, which are common postoperatively, many centres use iv magnesium sulphate 10 mmol iv over 20 minutes followed by 70 mmol iv over 24 hours to facilitate potassium correction.

REMOVAL OF LINES AND DRAINS

Chest drain (cardiac patients)

- Check for air leaks prior to drain removal and give iv analgesia prior to removal
- Remove drains when the hourly drainage is 20 ml/h or less for 5 hours consecutively

Central venous catheters

All cannulae are a potential source of infection and should be removed at the earliest possible opportunity, usually the second postoperative day. After this time peripheral cannulae are preferred. In patients who are unwell or have supraventricular tachycardia the central line may be left in for longer.

Pacing wires

Pacing wires can be removed as early as the third postoperative day provided the patient is haemodynamically stable, has normal electrolytes and has been in a stable rhythm and has not required pacing for the preceding 48 hours. If the INR is > 2.0 then warfarin must be omitted until the INR falls into the desired range. The postoperative instructions will include details of which wires are to be cut. Otherwise pull the wires. Pacing wires should draw out with minimal resistance. If there is resistance then do not pull harder. Prepare the site around the wire with aqueous Betadine, gently apply traction to the wire, apply more Betadine and cut it flush with the skin so that it retracts to below skin level.

Urinary catheters

Urinary catheters should be removed on the second postoperative day. For men with a history of significant prostatism it may be preferable to wait until they are more mobile and able to stand up to use a bottle.

Patients with epidural anaesthesia can have their catheters left in until the epidural is removed. For urinary retention leave the catheter in for 48 hours to rest the bladder and prescribe an α-blocker. If the patient goes into retention again they may require a long-term catheter and a referral to urology.

THE DETERIORATING PATIENT

As a basic principle, any deterioration in oxygen saturation, urine output, haemodynamic parameters, ECG or conscious level (including confusion), or inotrope requirements should be taken very seriously. The safest approach is to go back to first principles in assessing the problem. Assess the patient as you would an acute admission. First do an ABC check (airway, breathing, circulation). This will detect most life-threatening problems. Manage as appropriate (at an early stage, you should consult a senior colleague):

- Give oxygen and put in at least one large-bore iv cannula
- Take blood for FBC, U&E + creatinine + glucose and arrange a CXR
- While waiting for the blood results thoroughly reassess the patient including history and physical examination
- Check the blood gases and obtain data such as blood pressure, ECG, urine output and cardiac output studies (if available).

This process will detect most problems and lead to an appropriate diagnosis and management. Hypoxia is probably the most common problem and can lead to secondary cardiac failure.

COMPLICATIONS IN CARDIAC PATIENTS

POSTOPERATIVE BLEEDING

Postoperative bleeding is a serious problem. As a general rule chest tube drainage should be < 200 ml in the first hour and < 100 ml/h in subsequent hours. All bleeding comes from cut blood vessels thus anticoagulants and coagulopathies do not cause bleeding. Chest tube drainage of ≥ 200 ml prior to leaving the operating theatre may necessitate immediate re-exploration. Clotting factors, platelets and anti-fibrinolytic agents are not a substitute for this.

Drainage of > 200 ml/h is significant and requires investigation. A full clotting screen and platelet count is essential so that coagulopathies can be detected and corrected. A Hep-Con test will detect any unbound heparin and indicates bleeding which may stop with protamine. Blood product therapy with fresh frozen plasma and platelets can be effective when the clotting screen is abnormal but is not a substitute for operative haemostasis. Platelets may be required even in the presence of a normal platelet count due to platelet dysfunction caused by cardiopulmonary bypass or preoperative antiplatelet therapy. Fresh frozen plasma contains little fibrinogen and if plasma fibrinogen is low cryoprecipitate will be required. Trasylol is an anti-fibrinolytic agent that may slow bleeding and is usually given as a loading bolus followed by an infusion. The drainage usually decreases after the first hour.

Be aware of sudden drainage of a collection of blood. Pleural collections can suddenly drain quite large volumes (150–250 ml), particularly after moving or rolling the patient.

REOPENING FOR BLEEDING OR TAMPONADE

Signs of cardiac tamponade, increasing inotrope requirements or bleeding (>200 ml/h) are indications that surgical exploration may be necessary. Inform the consultant responsible immediately. Massive bleeding or severe haemodynamic compromise are indications for immediate reopening. Relieving an acute tamponade or stopping a major bleeding point can be life saving.

To reopen a chest:

- Call for senior help
- Whenever possible use full surgical aseptic technique; this may not always be possible
- Quickly paint the skin with Betadine
- Cut the skin and subcutaneous sutures with a scalpel or pair of scissors
- Grab the twist on the sternal wires and pull it up, cut the wire and pull it out (there are at least six wires but there may be as many as 12)
- For figure-of-eight wires cut the central 'x' where the wires cross and pull out both pieces of wire
- Open the chest and put in a retractor; this will usually lead to a rapid relief of tamponade and improvement in cardiac output and may be all that is necessary prior to arrival of a senior

- Be very careful of bypass grafts which may not be obvious at the front of the heart
- Finger pressure is usually sufficient to control an obvious bleeding point
- Replace lost volume

POSTOPERATIVE ARRHYTHMIAS

Bradycardia

- If causing haemodynamic compromise then pace the patient if pacing wires are in place
- If there are no pacing wires then consider atropine or an isoprenaline infusion
- If the bradycardia is persistent or compromising consult a cardiologist with regard to a temporary wire

Sinus tachycardia

This is usually encountered in patients who have been on β-blockers preoperatively. Reintroduce the β-blocker at a low dose provided the systemic blood pressure is adequate.

Supraventricular tachycardia

This is particularly common postoperatively and most units will have a protocol. Management depends on the presence or absence of haemodynamic compromise. For patients with a central line without compromise, amiodarone 5 mg/kg over 1 hour, followed by up to 900 mg by infusion over the ensuing 23 hours (with ECG monitoring) will rapidly slow the ventricular rate. This is followed up with oral amiodarone on the normal reducing schedule. If there is no central access, amiodarone can be given orally in a dose of 200 mg three times daily, for 1 week, 200 mg twice a day for the next week and 200 mg daily until review in the outpatient clinic in 6 weeks when it is usually stopped. An alternative is digoxin 500 μg iv by infusion slowly under ECG control, particularly if the patient was on digoxin preoperatively. Magnesium is a useful adjunct to this therapy and is given as a bolus of 10 mmol iv over 20 minutes followed by an infusion of 70 mmol of magnesium sulphate iv over 24 hours. It is important to correct the potassium to > 4.5 to improve the efficacy of magnesium. In the presence of haemodynamic compromise have a low threshold for emergency cardioversion.

Most patients will revert to sinus rhythm by the end of this protocol. If they still have narrow complex supraventricular tachycardia then add either atenolol or digoxin. These two drugs will only slow the ventricular response but not cause cardioversion. It is important to avoid the use of calcium-channel blockers and β-blockers in patients with a poor left ventricle.

POSTOPERATIVE HYPOTENSION

An adequate urine output is 0.5 ml/kg per hour. Higher urine outputs may be desirable in some patients, particularly in those with renal problems. Postoperative depletion of the intravascular space occurs as a result of bleeding, diuresis and third space fluid retention (accumulation of interstitial fluid) and leads to hypotension. Cardiopulmonary bypass leads to significant sodium and water retention postoperatively and so the fluid management of these patients is different from that of general surgical patients. In addition, the secretion of antidiuretic hormone and aldosterone as part of the normal physiological response to trauma leads to further sodium and water retention with concomitant potassium loss. Thus the principles of postoperative fluid management for these patients are:

- To restrict intravenous fluid and sodium input
- To give diuretics to help the excretion of excess sodium and water
- Potassium supplements and potassium-sparing diuretics may be used to avoid hypokalaemia

By avoiding the use of cardiopulmonary bypass, the physiological derangements of fluid and electrolyte balance are less severe than with conventional on-pump CABG, although those produced as part of the basic trauma response still occur. Fluid management is essentially the same as for a general surgical patient. Diuretics are not required unless the patient has been on diuretics preoperatively, in which case their preoperative diuretics can be continued.

History

The problem presents as oliguria (urine output < 0.5 ml/kg per hour), hypotension (fall in mean arterial pressure (MAP)) or a combination of both. Postoperative fluid management, as in other specialties, should consist of both maintenance (replacing essential losses, eg sweating, etc) and replacement (for an acquired deficit) fluid administration.

Intravenous fluids are usually discontinued on the second postoperative day when the patient is drinking adequately.

Examination

Clinical assessment is essential to avoid inappropriate fluid administration (risk of overload). Consider other causes of low BP and low urine output, eg cardiac failure, sepsis, hypothermia.

Initial treatment of an oliguric and hypovolaemic patient with diuretics will initially improve the urine output but at the cost of increasing the hypovolaemia. Lifting the patient's legs produces a quick and easily reversible auto transfusion. Hypotension due to underfilling improves within seconds of performing this manoeuvre.

Investigations

Daily weighing is invaluable in the monitoring of fluid balance and when the patient has regained their preoperative fluid status diuretics should be stopped. Patients who have been on diuretics preoperatively may require higher doses to achieve the desirable rate of weight loss and will probably require long-term postoperative diuretic therapy. Those not on diuretics have transient weight gain, but this is probably physiological and does not require specific treatment.

Treatment

Colloid volume replacement is the best method of correcting intravascular fluid deficits in small boluses of 100 ml. Administer the intravenous fluid and observe the CVP, pulmonary arterial pressure and MAP. No change in the CVP indicates severe hypovolaemia. A transient rise in the pressures and then a fall indicates relative hypovolaemia. With further boluses the pressures will show more of a sustained rise. When the pressures go up and stay up at an acceptable level the patient is euvolaemic. Similarly, for oliguria a colloid fluid given in boluses will lead to a rapid but appropriate restoration of circulating volume and urine production soon responds. If urine output fails to improve (> 0.5 ml/kg per hour) after adequate volume then urine output may respond to a small amount of diuretic (furosemide 20 mg iv).

POSTOPERATIVE ABDOMINAL COMPLICATIONS

Acute abdominal emergencies after cardiac surgery are rare but have very high mortality and morbidity. The main complications are bleeding from upper gastro-intestinal ulceration and intestinal ischaemia, which is generally due to impaired intestinal perfusion in patients with artherosclerosis of the mesenteric vasculature. Intestinal ischaemia may also occur as a result of embolism after valve surgery.

Constipation is a very common problem following surgery and commonly delays discharge or leads to readmission. All patients should receive mild laxatives until their bowels open.

Ischaemic bowel

In the anaesthetised patient abdominal signs are usually minimal and unreliable and so diagnosis and management depend upon a high index of clinical suspicion. Cardiovascular instability, increasing inotrope requirements, unexplained metabolic acidosis and leukocytosis are all possible signs but the absence of one or more of these signs does not exclude the diagnosis. it is important to have a low threshold for seeking the opinion of an experienced general surgeon. Emergency laparotomy and resection of affected intestinal segments may be life saving. Extubated patients can usually provide an adequate history and clinical examination for a diagnosis to be made. The clinical signs of ischaemic bowel may not be as dramatic as the symptoms and degree of physiological upset. This is partly explained by ischaemia starting submucosally whereas abdominal signs become significant only when serosal involvement occurs. However, prompt investigation and surgical intervention are still needed.

Bleeding ulcer

For bleeding the management includes:

- Replacement of intravascular volume
- Reversal of warfarin if appropriate
- Gastric mucosal protection with a PPI
- Early diagnosis by urgent endoscopy
- Emergency surgery if appropriate medical therapy fails or if there is re-bleeding

POSTOPERATIVE PYREXIA

Normal body temperature is 36.7–37°C orally and 37.3–37.6°C rectally and tympanic membrane temperature probes are equivalent to rectal temperature. There is a circadian rhythm for body temperature with normal temperature being higher in the evening. Seventy-five per cent of cardiac surgical patients will develop postoperative pyrexia. The most common causes are atelectasis, respiratory tract infections, superficial wound infections, infection of indwelling lines and urinary tract infections.

Generally pyrexia of less than 38.9°C rectal or 38.3°C oral is benign in origin and will settle with appropriate surgical management and antibiotic therapy. Pyrexias greater than this are more likely to be serious. Similarly, pyrexia after the fourth postoperative day has a high probability of being serious in nature. Management consists of a thorough clinical evaluation to determine the likely source of infection. Specimens should be obtained for microbiological examination, and antibiotic therapy may be started empirically and changed in the light of clinical progress and antibiotic sensitivities.

POSTOPERATIVE HYPERTENSION

Sublingual calcium-channel blockers should be avoided as the effect is unpredictable and may precipitate a significant fall in blood pressure. In the early postoperative period most patients have a low BP and seldom require their antihypertensive medication. As pressure increases postoperatively antihypertensive medication should be reintroduced at the lowest dose and increased as clinically indicated. In patients with a history of myocardial infarction are usually prescribed β-blocker. Patients with impaired ventricular function benefit from ACE inhibitors. It is important to avoid prescribing β-blockers and calcium-channel antagonists together.

RESPIRATORY FAILURE

COMMON CAUSES OF POSTOPERATIVE RESPIRATORY FAILURE

- Atelectasis
- Pulmonary oedema
- Bronchopneumonia
- Pneumothorax

The diagnosis is based on clinical history, examination, CXR and ABG. Administer oxygen, treat the underlying cause and, if necessary, get an opinion from an anaesthetist. Senior colleagues should certainly be advised. If oxygen via a normal face mask is not sufficient go to Hi-Flow oxygen. If 100% oxygen via Hi-Flow is insufficient then the patient may need continuous positive airways pressure (CPAP). A patient likely to need CPAP should have an anaesthetic opinion as a significant number of these patients go on to require intubation.

PUMP PSYCHOSIS (ACUTE PARANOID PSYCHOSIS)

Acute paranoid psychosis typically occurs 3–4 days after surgery and, though not exclusive to cardiac surgery, does occur more commonly than in other surgical specialties.

History

The first signs are agitation, usually in the evening, and progress to acute paranoid psychosis in the early hours of the morning. Preoperative psychiatric history, alcoholism, postoperative complications, sleep deprivation and opioid analgesics are risk factors.

Examination

In particular look for hypoxia. Turn the lights on and put the patient in a quiet, well-lit room where they can be constantly observed. Noise, darkness, reflections and shadows cause disorientation and hallucinations. If possible, try to persuade the patient to take haloperidol until the desired level of control is achieved, since they can harm themselves and others.

Investigations

Once they are sufficiently co-operative give oxygen and investigate thoroughly for any underlying medical or surgical cause in particular respiratory failure, infection, heart failure.

Treatment

The principal aims of treatment are to sedate the patient sufficiently to prevent exhaustion and to identify any underlying physiological or metabolic cause. The best management is to recognise the problem in its early stages and prevent further deterioration. For the agitated patient give oxygen and initiate treatment with haloperidol IM or IV and then investigate the cause. The haloperidol can be repeated until the desired degree of control is achieved. In severely psychotic patients a higher initial dose may be necessary. Adequate treatment with haloperidol will usually make the patient suitable for full clinical examination and investigation to determine any underlying cause.

STERNAL WOUND PROBLEMS

A clicking sternum in isolation, without signs of infection, is not in itself a significant problem. However, underlying infection must be vigorously excluded. A superficial wound infection will usually settle after the wound has been opened adequately and the pus allowed to drain. A serosanguineous leakage from the chest wound is often benign but can herald wound dehiscence and so must be treated seriously. It occurs due to a communication between the pericardium and the skin. If this occurs in the presence of signs of infection then consider mediastinitis.

Infection or discharge in the presence of sternal instability is a very serious problem since the sternal instability may be a product of a deep infection. Further radiological investigation, surgical exploration and rewiring may be necessary. Sternal dehiscence is usually a consequence of mediastinitis. The treatment is difficult and the mortality high. Early diagnosis and appropriate intervention are essential. Of particular concern are mediastinitis and valve infections. For patients with abnormal or prosthetic heart valves postoperative bacterial endocarditis is rare (0.5–1.5%) but potentially fatal. Multiple blood cultures and appropriate antibiotic therapy after discussion with microbiology are essential. Echocardiography is a diagnostic aid but is unlikely to demonstrate typical findings of endocarditis in the early stages post operatively. In suspected cases antibiotic therapy should not be delayed by waiting for an echocardiogram or microbiology results.

CARDIOTHORACIC TRAUMA

The mode of injury is essential to the understanding of these injuries and their management. Blunt thoracic trauma is responsible for the majority of cardiothoracic trauma and is most frequently treated conservatively apart from the judicious use of chest drains.

Penetrating trauma patients need to be assessed quickly as deterioration can occur extremely quickly and the management frequently involves emergency surgery.

BLUNT TRAUMA

History

The spectrum of injury following blunt chest trauma is extremely broad, ranging from minor chest wall bruising and uncomplicated rib fracture to massive chest wall injury with multiple rib fractures and extensive disruption of major intra thoracic structures. Common modes of injury include falls from a height and road traffic accidents. The history of the impact particularly the velocity is important in evaluating the likelihood of serious internal injuries.

Examination

Assessment should follow the ABC pattern as for any major injury. While there may be external evidence of chest wall injury such as bruising of rib fractures, it is imporatnt to have a high index of suspicion for major intrathoracic injury.

Investigations

A chest X-ray is an extremely valuable aid to the diagnosis of chest trauma problems. Important points to look for include, the presence of a widened mediastinum, fracture of the first rib, pneumothorax, haemothorax, diaphragmatic rupture, hernia or a flail segment. CT thorax may also be necessary as it allows for assessment of lung parenchyma for contusion, the great vessels for transection/dissection (with contrast), associated abdominal injury and cervical spine assessment.

Treatment

It is important to appreciate the severity of injury and the number of organ systems affected. As with any trauma, ALS and ATLS provide a guide for initial assessment and resuscitation. With rib bruising and fracture it is essential to achieve adequate pain relief as early as possible to avoid atelectasis and infection, particularly in smokers. This can be achieved by simple oral analgesia but this should be escalated to iv (patient-controlled analgesia) and even epidural/nerve block to achieve a pain-free respiratory cycle. In the setting of deteriorating blood gases with poor ventilation, contusion or flail segment, positive pressure ventilation may be necessary and some patients need intubation.

It is important to have a low threshold for chest drain insertion, as any pneumothorax is likely to enlarge and may contain some blood. This is mandatory in those that end up having positive pressure ventilation. A large air leak despite adequate position of a large drain should raise the possibility of a major airway or lung injury.

In the presence of hypotension, elevated jugular venous pressure and muffled heart sounds cardiac tamponade needs to be ruled out. If the diagnosis is in question or the clinical condition permits some delay, echocardiogram should be done to allow guided drainage. However, this is seldom the case and needle aspiration is necessary as a diagnostic and therapeutic procedure.

PENETRATING TRAUMA

This is thankfully rare in the UK and so is infrequently encountered. These injuries can be relatively minor if limited to skin, muscle or subcutaneous tissue and are often dealt with entirely by A&E if the CXR is completely normal.

Thoracic services are often called to admit patients who have had chest stabbings with a resulting pneumothorax with or without haemothorax from the chest wall vasculature. These patients generally need a chest drain to re-inflate the lung and drain any blood (second drain). If the chest drainage is limited and there is minimal air leak, these patients respond well to conservative therapy with antibiotics, analgesia and drainage. Suspicion of a visceral injury in a stable patient necessitates future imaging to assess the heart, great vessels, lung parenchyma and any extra-thoracic injury. These may require urgent repair depending on the pattern of injury.

An unstable patient with a high index of suspicion for thoracic rather than abdominal injuries (penetration injury above the nipple line with no abdominal signs) may require immediate transfer to theatre for thoracotomy. Occasionally patients present with penetrating injury to the chest with no output (pulseless). ATLS guidelines support the use of emergency thoracotomy in A&E in this setting to allow for cardiac massage, tamponade decompression and aortic cross clamping. This is a difficult procedure that can be time consuming in those not used to performing thoracotomies. These patients often have an undefined period of arrest and have a dire prognosis. However, occasional successes occur.

It is important in the inevitable stress of such a scenario to attend carefully to the ABCs while the decisions/logistics of thoracotomy are being explored. This invariably means:

- Endotracheal intubation
- Large-bore iv access for drug and resuscitation fluid
- Rhythm assessment for a shockable rhythm

If thoracotomy is contemplated time is of the essence. In the absence of a great deal of experience lateral thoracotomy is recommended. This entails:

- Scalpel incision in the fourth or fifth intercostal space (nipple) through the intercostal space into the pleura
- The incision can now be extended anteriorly or posteriorly (or both) as needed
- Once inside the chest insert the rib retractor to separate the ribs as much as possible
- After brief inspection the most rewarding procedure is to open the pericardium parallel to the phrenic nerve to aid diagnosis and drainage of tamponade, assessment of the location of any cardiac injuries and allow internal massage
- It is worthwhile pausing after a few minutes of massage to assess rhythm, as internal defibrillation can be more effective than external paddles

There is little consensus for emergency thoracotomy. Some advocate the use of balloon catheters to occlude any cardiac injuries manually while other favour deep mattress sutures (pericardial pledgets). In the absence of cardiac injury massage should continue until spontaneous output is restored. The thoracotomy and compressions should not distract from ongoing drug administration as per ALS, and compression should only stop for rhythm checks. Wall suction will allow visualisation of most of the heart and lung on that side. If there has been substantial blood loss or initial efforts have been unfruitful some advocate the use of aortic cross clamping to increase afterload on the heart and improve cerebral perfusion. If no injury is seen at left lateral thoracotomy, the contralateral chest or abdomen may be opened but at this stage little can be achieved.

CHAPTER 7

NEUROSURGERY

M O MURPHY AND M MURPHY

Many newly qualified doctors are afraid of neurosurgical issues and few will pursue a career in neurosurgery. However, neurosurgical conditions are relatively ubiquitous, with head injuries often managed by an array of specialties, including A&E, general surgery and orthopaedics, in regional and district hospitals. It is therefore important for all junior doctors to have a good understanding of the neurosurgical 'basics'. Much of what is written for this audience aims to give the reader a comprehensive understanding of the subject, without addressing some of the practical issues of caring for a neurosurgical patient.

GLASGOW COMA SCORE

The Glasgow Coma Score (GCS) is a reliable, reproducible measure of a patient's consciousness level. The GCS is scored between 3 (worst) and 15 (best) and consists of three parameters: best motor response, best verbal response, best eye response.

MOTOR RESPONSE

Does the patient obey commands? If not, what is his or her motor response to pain? It is the **best** motor response of the arms (not legs) which is taken. Do not use the sternal rub as this makes it impossible to distinguish between localising and flexing. Pain applied to the supraorbital ridge is therefore preferable.

VERBAL RESPONSE

How coherent is the patient's verbal effort?

EYE OPENING

The degree of stimulation required to cause the patient to open their eyes.

Each component in the GCS is scored according to Table 7.1 and the total added to give a final score ranging from 3(min) to 15(max).

Table 7.1 Glasgow Coma Score

		Score
Motor response	• Obeys commands – will perform simple tasks on request	6
	• Localising – hand comes up over the body to brush away the examiner	5
	• Normal flexion – hand comes up over the body but fails to progress above the shoulders	4
	• Abnormal flexion – spastic movement of the fists upwards and inwards	3
	• Extension – wrists and arms turn down and move away from the body	2
	• None – no movement in spite of supraorbital pain which causes half of the nail bed to blanche	1
Verbal response	• Orientated	5
	• Confused/ disorientated – fluent but disorientated speech in sentences	4
	• Inappropriate words – coherent words or short phrases in inappropriate context	3
	• Incomprehensible sounds – noise or groans, but no words	2
	• None	1
Eyes opening	• Spontaneously – patient spontaneously looks about	4
	• To speech – patient opens eyes only on request	3
	• To pain – painful stimuli cause the patient to open eyes	2
	• None – will not open eyes even in the presence of significant central pain	1

Neurosurgeons prefer to be given a breakdown of a patient's consciousness level in words not numbers, ie eye-opening to pain, localising with incomprehensible sounds. This is a better description of the patient's condition than a number. In addition, it convinces them that an accurate assessment of the patient has been made.

The GCS should be a report of the best motor response, best verbal response and best eye opening, meaning that if during the course of an examination several different responses are ascertained, then only the best should be recorded. This is quite distinct from the situation where a clear deterioration occurs over time. In severe head injuries remember to evaluate and record the GCS prior to intubation.

Normally, the pupils are equal and reactive to light and the pupillary size and reactivity are often mentioned along with the GCS. If the pupils become fixed and dilated the patient has 'coned' and urgent action must be taken if a surgically remediable lesion is present. Once paralysed for intubation the patient's pupils should be closely observed. Where the patient has been intubated and ventilated and is inaccessible to neurological examination, the pupils are the only reliable way of detecting a deterioration.

Dysphasia may be expressive and/or receptive and may be the result of a focal lesion of Broca's and/or Wernicke's areas respectively, or it may be secondary to a global dominant hemisphere lesion. A global dysphasia or aphasia may result in the patient having a motor response of localising and no verbal response in spite of being very alert and opening the eyes spontaneously.

HEAD INJURY

Head injury is a common A&E presentation and most commonly affected are young, fit men. Incorrect evaluation or inappropriate management of a head injury may result in needless death or debility in this patient group. **Primary** brain injury is incurred at the time of impact whereas secondary injury arises later due to hypoxia, raised intracerebral pressure, cerebral oedema and infection. Management of head trauma predominantly aims to minimise **secondary** brain injury.

MILD HEAD INJURY

Defined as GCS of > 12. This group of patients is at risk of being mismanaged if history or examination is inadequate. These patients may present without a convincing history, they look dishevelled, often smell of alcohol and frequently cause trouble in A&E. Hence, often the early features of serious injury are falsely ascribed to a drunken or drugged state.

Some patients with mild head injury are at significant risk of deterioration from an intracranial haematoma. It is therefore important to be able to screen these patients effectively into high- and low-risk categories. The most salient features of patients at risk in this category are:

- Presence of a skull fracture
- Presence of confusion
- Depression in consciousness level

In the presence of a skull fracture and either of the other two features the patient has a high chance of having an intracranial haematoma, and should therefore proceed directly to CT scanning (Table 7.2).

Table 7.2 Head injuries – when to take a CT scan

Presence of a skull fracture	Presence of confusion	Likelihood of clot
−	−	1/6000
−	+	1/120
+	−	1/32
+	+	1/4

MODERATE HEAD INJURY

This is defined by a GCS of 8–12. The same principles apply as for mild head injury. However, with these patients the key decision-making issue is when to intubate and when to refer to neurosurgery. If in doubt whether to intubate, have an anaesthetist evaluate the patient. All moderate head injuries should have a CT scan and at least be discussed with a neurosurgical team.

SEVERE HEAD INJURY

Severe head injury is defined as GCS < 8. Common mechanisms of injury include road traffic accidents, falls from height and assault. Frequently these patients have polytrauma and are brought to the A&E resuscitation area. It is important to discern those with isolated neurosurgical issues from those with multisystem problems.

Examination

After assessment of ABCs, record each component of the GCS on a neurological observation chart and note whether the pupils are equal and reactive. It is very important to inspect the entire head for signs of a laceration, bruise/haematoma, puncture site or signs of a base of skull fracture.

Investigations

In the A&E setting the following represent the minimum investigations, which should be performed as soon as possible: an FBC, U&E, coagulation, group and save, X-rays of lateral cervical spine, pelvis, chest (these three constitute the trauma screen) and any other clinically indicated radiology. The next stage is to decide whether the head injury is isolated or not, which in practice is achieved by a skeletal survey. It is important to take a CT scan of the brain as early as the patient's condition allows.

Treatment

Non-isolated severe head injury

With all trauma the first concern should always be for the patient's cardiorespiratory welfare. Once the 'ABCs' have been evaluated and stabilised, immobilise the cervical spine with collar, sandbags and tape. Call the anaesthetist if the patient is not already intubated. If a laparotomy or thoracotomy is indicated this should precede neurosurgical referral. Once haemodynamically stable, evaluate the patient by CT scanning. When referring the patient to a neurosurgeon, describe all of the patient's injuries and if accepted for transfer send all imaging with the patient, including those pertinent to other injuries.

Isolated severe head injury

If the head injury is isolated a CT scan is required. Prior to scanning ask yourself if the patient needs to be intubated (almost certainly! – see box on page 268) and whether they would benefit from mannitol (see below). When the CT has been performed a neurosurgical opinion should be sought.

If pupils are fixed and dilated give 200 ml of 20% mannitol. This is an osmotic diuretic that temporarily reduces intracranial pressure (ICP). If the patient becomes agitated, this should first be treated with haloperidol and analgesia. Continued agitation is reason to consider intubation.

Treat with a non-sedating analgesic. The strongest and most useful analgesic is dihydrocodeine (orally or intramuscularly). Do not use sedating analgesics or diazepam unless you intend to intubate and ventilate the patient for a scan as these may precipitate a false deterioration in GCS. Haloperidol is very effective and underused in the management of agitation.

If the patient cones it is essential to intubate and ventilate the patient if not already done. Give 200 ml 20% mannitol, scan the patient and update the neurosurgical team.

WHEN TO INTUBATE?

- When the motor response is flexing or worse
- When the patient is unable to maintain an airway
- When an extremely rapid deterioration from a good consciousness level has occurred
- When the patient has agitation refractory to pharmacological measures
- When there is failure of pharmacological attempts to control seizures

---

INFORMATION REQUIRED WHEN REFERRING A SEVERE HEAD INJURY

- Patient name and age (if available)
- Mechanism and time of injury
- Consciousness level prior to intubation (include any changes in GCS)
- State of the pupils + any changes
- Focal neurological deficit (even if minor/transient)
- Seizures
- Headache/nausea/vomiting
- Presence of confusion depressed level of consciousness or a skull fracture

POSSIBLE CT FINDINGS

- Extradural haematoma
- Subdural haematoma
- Contusions/intracerebral haematoma
- Fracture ± depressed
- Diffuse axonal injury
- Mixture of the above
- Normal

OMINOUS OCCURRENCES IN HEAD INJURIES

- ↓GCS
- Fixing/dilating pupil
- The Cushing response of ↑BP, ↓heart rate, ↓respiration
- Seizures

Unless the diagnosis is known and treatment underway, any of these developments necessitates the need for another scan

READING A CT BRAIN SCAN

CT is the most useful radiological investigation in significant head injury. When looking at CT films, ask yourself four questions:

- Is the midline in the midline or is there asymmetry? If there is a mass lesion the midline is pushed **away** from the side of the lesion
- Is there blood in the subarachnoid space/around the circle of Willis? (Classically in the shape of a star at the base of the brain)
- Is there also hydrocephalus?
  - Plump lateral ventricles
  - Round third ventricle
  - ↑ Periventricular lucency (the brain around the ventricles is blacker than the brain distant from the ventricles due to trans-ependymal flow of CSF from the ventricles, under pressure into the brain)
  - ↑ Visible surface sulci

- Is there abnormal whiteness (indicates fresh blood)? This is most easily appreciated by comparing both hemispheres:

  - Intracerebral (within brain, away from dural surface)?
  - Extradural (homogeneous, bright white and concave shape)?
  - Subdural (convex shape)?
  - Contusion (within the cortex, but inhomogeneous, usually at surface)?
  - Tumour (heterogeneous, may not be clearly visible)?

READING THE CT SCAN

- CSF is black
- Bone/calcium and **fresh** blood are **white**
- Subdural collections are convex from the outside, ie they look like a crescentic moon
- Extradural collections are concave from the outside

CSF LEAKS

After trauma there are generally two types of CSF leak, and both are associated with fractured base of skull: CSF otorrhoea (leakage from the ear), and CSF rhinorrhoea (leakage from the nose), which indicate that there is also a route for microbe entry (Table 7.3). The patient is therefore at risk of meningitis while CSF is leaking. These patients must be observed for signs of meningitis in a hospital setting until the leak stops and the patient must not be discharged if actively leaking CSF. If the leak does not stop, surgery may be indicated.

Table 7.3 Distinguishing features of skull fractures

Fracture of anterior cranial fossa	Fracture of middle cranial fossa
CSF otorrhoea ± deafness Battle's sign (mastoid bruising)	CSF rhinorrhoea Panda (raccoon) eyes Subconjunctival haemorrhage ± anosmia ± facial weakness

CLEARING THE SPINE OF A HEAD-INJURED PATIENT

Assessing the cervical spine and associated injuries requires a full history and physical assessment. Multiple trauma patients, unconscious patients or patients with neck pain following injury have a cervical spine injury until proved otherwise. Normal findings in cervical spine X-rays do not exclude a spinal injury and a clinical assessment is mandatory.

The cervical spine series of X-rays consists of AP, lateral and open mouth views. A minimum of a lateral cervical spine film showing C1 to the top of T1 is required unless the mechanism does not suggest neck injury and the patient is completely lucid and has no neck pain/tenderness or limitation in range of motion. The goal of management is to identify the patients with an injury (Table 7.4), and to prevent the development/deterioration of neurological symptoms.

CERVICAL SPINE X-RAYS

- Check that the X-ray is of the patient you are dealing with
- Lateral X-rays should include C1–T1. If you cannot see the C7–T1 junction the film is inadequate, and further imaging is required. Look at the lateral cervical spine X-ray for vertebral line, posterior vertebral line, and spinolaminar line (Figure 7.1)
- AP view should include the spinous processes of C2–T1
- Open mouth views should visualise the entire odontoid process, and the lateral masses. (This view is not possible in intubated patients, and CT of C1–C3 is usually indicated)
- Swimmer's views of shoulder pull-down views can be used to image the lower cervical spine/thoracic spine junction

---

Cervical spine protection, along with airway control, is the first priority in management of the multiple trauma patient. However, clearance of the cervical spine is not the immediate priority. If a patient requires urgent surgery and cannot be fully worked-up for cervical spine injury, the collar is left in situ and full spinal precautions apply. The spine can be cleared later when the patient is stable.

Table 7.4 Abnormalities on cervical spine X-ray

Physiological lordosis	Normal anterior curvature – absence may indicate subtle injury
Vertebral alignment	Assess for subluxations/fracture dislocations
	The anterior vertebral line, posterior vertebral line and spinolaminar line should be smooth lines, no steps. A step in the posterior vertebral line is more significant. Translation of > 3.5 mm is significant
	Anterior subluxation of one vertebra on the one below suggests facet dislocation (< 50% of the width of the vertebra subluxed suggests unifacet dislocation; > 50%, bifacet subluxation)
Vertebral bodies	Compression/burst-type injuries. Below C2, vertebral bodies are square shaped. Compression fractures result in anterior wedging or tear-drop fractures of anterior inferior body
Disc height	Loss of height indicates disc herniation – usually posteriorly
Spinous processes	Look at the spinous processes for fractures (clay-shoveller's fracture at C7)
Prevertebral tissue shadow	The soft-tissue shadow anterior to the cervical spine formed by the pharynx above C4, and posterior larynx and oesophagus below C4. Above C4, width < 50% the width of the vertebra. Below C4 width should be equal to vertebral body width. An increase suggests haematoma caused by fracture
Atlanto-occipital junction	Rarely get atlanto-occipital dislocation (C0 fracture). Distance between atlas and occiput should not exceed 5 mm
Atlanto-dens interval	Suggests rupture of transverse ligament and should not exceed 3 mm

Figure 7.1 Normal lateral cervical spine X-ray showing the anterior, spinolaminar and posterior columns

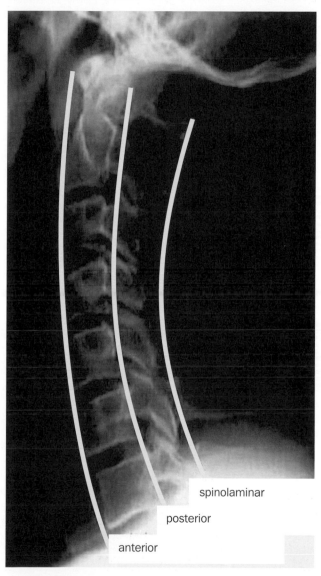

spinolaminar

posterior

anterior

Clinical clearance

An alert and conscious patient with no neurological signs but with neck pain requires radiological assessment including AP, lateral and open mouth views. If these show normal findings, a clinical assessment should be performed.

Patients can be clinically cleared and do not require cervical spine imaging provided that they fulfil all of the following criteria:

- No neck pain
- Alert and conscious (GCS 15/15)
- Not under the influence of drugs/alcohol
- Neurologically normal
- No painful distracting injuries or facial fractures
- No tenderness on palpating the neck
- Normal, pain-free active range of motion

Radiological clearance (Figure 7.2)

If there is severe localised neck pain or X-rays are suspicious, a CT scan of the level in question should be done. Most neurosurgical and many non-neurosurgical units now use 3D-reconstructed CT scanning of the cervical spine as standard trauma neck imaging. Any patient with a neurological deficit must be assumed to have an underlying spinal injury, and treated with full spinal precautions. X-rays are mandatory, as is further imaging in the form of CT/MRI. Urgent specialist review should be sought.

In an unconscious patient, one must assume a cervical spine injury. Normal findings in cervical spine X-rays do not exclude an injury. The hard collar must be left in situ until the patient can be clinically assessed. If the patient is likely to be comatose for a prolonged period, an MR scan and clearance by an orthopaedic or neuro surgeon is indicated.

Spinal boards

The spinal board is used for the transfer of patients to the A&E department. It is not a treatment for a spinal injury, and can lead to serious decubitus ulcers with prolonged usage. Patients with suspected spinal injuries should be log rolled and examined during the ATLS assessment – the spinal board is removed, and the patient immobilised on a firm bed until radiological assessment.

Figure 7.2 Algorithm for radiological clearance of spine in the head-injured patient

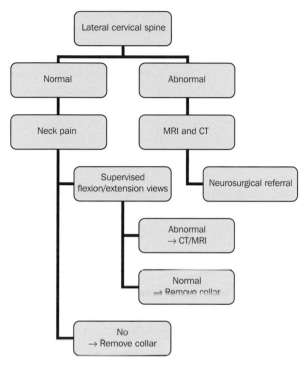

MANAGEMENT

See Table 7.5.

Table 7.5 Management of cervical spine injury

Immobilise	Protect the spine at all times until injury can be excluded – use hard collar, sandbags and tape. Spinal board for transport
Airway	If a patient requires intubation for airway support, this should be carried out maintaining the neck in a neutral position and preventing movement

Continued

Table 7.5 *Continued*

Intravenous access and fluids	Large-bore iv × 2, iv fluids may be required in the quadriplegic patient as they can suffer from neurogenic shock. (Loss of cardiac sympathetic tone causing bradycardia and hypotension.) Hypotension in the trauma patient must be assumed to be hypovolaemic initially, and they should be treated with fluid resuscitation. Urinary output (via a catheter) can help to distinguish
Steroids	High-dose methylprednisolone has fallen out of favour and should not be used
Refer	**Urgent review**

COMPOUND DEPRESSED SKULL FRACTURE

This is defined as a laceration overlying a skull fracture, where the outer table of the bony fragment is at least as depressed as the inner table of the normal cranium. The likelihood of an intracranial clot is high after such a head injury.

MANAGEMENT

These injuries are usually due to assault resulting in a penetrating head injury

- If the weapon is still present do not remove it
- Ensure there are no other wounds first (head and body)
- Shave the skin around the laceration
- Remove any **free** foreign objects
- Clean the wound
- Suture the wound for haemostasis

Definitive treatment is in a neurosurgical setting, where debridement and elevation can be performed.

BONE FLAP INFECTION

History

This presents in a patient who has previously had a neurosurgical procedure (craniotomy).

Examination

The patient has a boggy, fluctuant wound, pus discharge, ↓GCS, seizures.

Investigations

CT with contrast to define any possible intracranial extension.

Treatment

Removal of the bone flap, and give antibiotics. It is essential to swab the wound before starting antibiotics. It is important to recognise this potential complication and discuss suspected cases with a neurosurgeon.

CHRONIC SUBDURAL HAEMATOMA

History

Chronic subdural haematoma (CSDH) usually occurs in older patients, half of whom have a history of minor head injury in the immediately preceding weeks. The patients are often conscious at the time of presentation and frequently are on warfarin or aspirin. Headache occurs as a consequence of raised intracranial pressure. Patients may also develop seizures.

Examination

Assess for focal neurological defect with confusion.

Treatment

CSDHs are drained by burr holes when there are symptoms or a mass effect is seen on CT scan. It is essential for coagulation to be normalised prior to surgery. CSDHs have a relatively good prognosis, even in elderly patients.

SUBARACHNOID HAEMORRHAGE

Subarachnoid haemorrhage (SAH) is defined as intracranial bleeding in the subarachnoid plane. Spontaneous SAH is usually due to rupture of a Berry aneurysm. No matter how well a patient with a SAH appears do not assume that this is anything but a potentially lethal condition.

It is important to appreciate that patients with SAH can re-bleed and die at any time, hence the importance of prompt investigation and diagnosis in these patients. Once a diagnosis of SAH is reached refer to a neurosurgical unit as the prognosis of SAH can be dismal.

History

Headache with loss of consciousness, collapse or sudden death. The headache of SAH is very characteristic:

- Sudden onset of very severe headache
- Often associated with photophobia
- Often associated with nausea and vomiting

Examination

- Neck stiffness (ie meningism) ± focal neurological deficit

Investigations (Figure 7.3)

- Check ABG (oxygenation, carbon dioxide level)
- CT scan (for hydrocephalus or re-bleed)
- Check Na^+ daily (minimum) as these patients are at significant risk of hyponatraemia (due to the cerebral salt-wasting syndrome (CSWS))

Treatment

In managing SAH it is important to have a good understanding of the possible complications, with an appreciation of how best to minimise these:

- Strict, flat bed rest
- Neurological observations should be performed, and documented every 2 hours and a senior should be informed of any deterioration
- Keep well hydrated (supplement with iv infusion if necessary – use 0.9% saline)

Figure 7.3 Investigation algorithm for subarachnoid haemorrhage

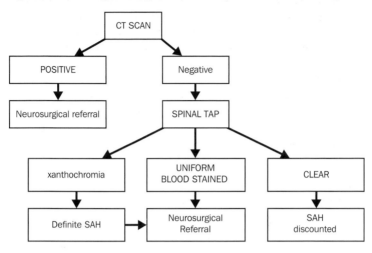

- Keep well oxygenated (hypoxia increases risk of infarction secondary to vasospasm)
- Give nimodipine 60 mg 4 hourly (given PO/iv/NG (nasogastric) to minimise risk of cerebral infarction secondary to vasospasm)
- Watch BP. Do not treat hypertension unless systolic BP > 200 mmHg and diastolic BP >120 mmHg, and then treat with small doses of sublingual nifedipine (eg 5 mg) after consultation with local neurosurgeon
- Give regular laxatives (straining increases intracranial pressure)

Table 7.6 The lumbar puncture

Indications	Contraindications
Diagnosis of SAH in cases where CT is normal	Unsure why it is being done
Rule-out meningitis	Any midline shift on the scan
(differential diagnosis: CT −ve SAH)	Any asymmetry in the ventricular system
Treat communicating hydrocephalus (on the instruction of a neurosurgeon)	A space-occupying lesion
Diagnose malignant meningitis	Non-communicating hydrocephalus

Table 7.7 Natural history of untreated SAH

Out of 100 patients:	15 die before hospital
Leaving 85:	15 die within 24 hours
Leaving 70:	15 die within 2 weeks
Leaving 55:	15 die within 2 months
Leaving 40:	15 die within 2 years
Leaving 25:	Alive at 2 years

SPINAL DISEASE

CERVICAL SPINE

Degenerative disease of the cervical spine

Cervical spine degenerative disease has two main patterns of presentation: radiculopathy or myelopathy. Radiculopathy is characterised by shooting pains down the arm, which may be associated with motor, reflex or sensory changes. The distribution of these changes relates to the compressed nerve root.

Myelopathy is caused by central disc herniation in the cervical spine and results in compression of the nerves to the legs and arms, if the lesion is high enough. This manifests as an upper motor neurone lesion. In these instances the patient usually reports frequent episodes of legs 'giving way'. In cases of cervical cord compression causing a myelopathy, investigation and treatment should be more prompt than for those with just a radiculopathy, as progression of a myelopathy may result in paraplegia.

Non-degenerative disease of the cervical spine

In general, the degree of urgency of investigation is dictated by the degree and speed of progression of the deficit. These cases may present with cauda equina syndrome. Causes:

- Tumour (often secondary spread)
- Disc
- Epidural haematoma/abscess (inflammatory indices ↑)

THE LUMBAR SPINE

Degenerative disease of the lumbar spine presents in one of two patterns:

- Cauda equina syndrome
- Radiculopathy

Note: low back pain alone is seldom treatable by surgery.

The cauda equina is formed by nerve roots caudal to the level of spinal cord termination. Cauda equina syndrome may result from any lesion that compresses cauda equina nerve roots and is defined as low back pain, unilateral or usually bilateral sciatica, saddle sensory disturbances, bladder and bowel dysfunction, and variable lower extremity motor and sensory loss. Cauda equina syndrome is discussed on pages 281–283.

LUMBAR SPINAL DISEASE

Lumbar radiculopathy

This is due to lateral disc herniation. It presents with unilateral leg pain ± neurological deficit. This pain is often referred to as 'sciatica'. The natural history of this condition is such that a third progress, a third wax and wane, and a third get better. Therefore, unless there are features of cauda equina syndrome, radiculopathy should be treated as a non-emergency. Preliminary management involves NSAIDs, rest and physiotherapy.

CAUDA EQUINA SYNDROME

History

This is usually an acute presentation as a result of central, lumbar disc herniation. It presents with acute lower back pain and:

- Unilateral or bilateral leg pain ± motor and/or sensory neurological deficit
- Sphincter impairment – bladder and bowel dysfunction
- Perineal (saddle) + perianal paraesthesia

Examination

There may be local tenderness over the lower back with loss or reduction of lower limb reflexes. Note that hyperactive reflexes suggest spinal cord involvement and exclude the diagnosis of cauda equina syndrome. There may be a reduction in light touch sensation over the perineum 'saddle' area. Anal sphincter tone is characteristically diminished. There may be evidence of urinary retention or a large residual volume on bladder catheterisation.

Figure 7.4 Dermatome map

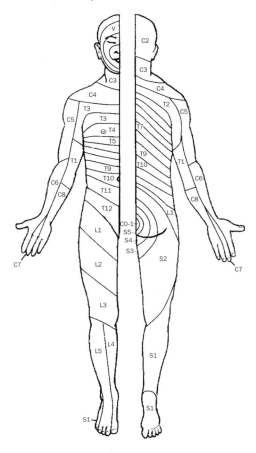

Treatment

It is important to recognise this condition and expedite urgent investigation and transfer to a neurosurgical unit because the greater the extent and duration of the lesion, the more likely the patient is to suffer permanent foot drop, bowel, bladder and sexual dysfunction – this condition affects the young and active population.

Investigations should include an MRI (optimally) or a CT and an urgent neurosurgical referral should be made.

CNS TUMOURS

'Brain tumours' encompass a very wide range of pathologies, with varying degrees of malignancy and prognoses. The presentation of brain tumours is with one/any combination of raised ICP, focal neurological deficit, seizures and decreased consciousness level.

History

It is important to ascertain whether the patient could have a cancer elsewhere, ie might this be a secondary? It is also important to ascertain their cardiorespiratory status and whether there are any seizures.

Investigations

MRI is the investigation of choice although a CT scan with and without contrast is usually sufficient to at least make a diagnosis.

Treatment

Referral to a neurosurgical unit should be prompt but not urgent unless the patient is unconscious or deteriorating rapidly. The patient should be started on dexamethasone (with a gastro-protective agent) to reduce peri-lesion oedema and reduce the patient's symptoms.

Hydrocephalus is defined as ventricular dilatation associated with raised intracranial pressure. There are two types: communicating and non-communicating.

Communicating hydrocephalus is where the entire ventricular system is enlarged, including the fourth ventricle. Typical features include a round third ventricle and sausage-shaped enlargement of the lateral ventricles. Periventricular lucency may be increased as evidenced by darker appearance of the white matter around the ventricles on CT scan.

Non-communicating hydrocephalus is caused by blockage at one point, causing proximal hydrocephalus. This occurs most commonly at the aqueduct of Sylvius, the narrowest part of the ventricular system and results in dilatation of both lateral and the third ventricles. In this case the fourth ventricle is normal/small.

Examination

This depends on the duration of onset and patient's age. Paediatric patients with chronic hydrocephalus demonstrate failure to thrive and mental retardation. If the onset is more acute they can demonstrate irritability, impaired consciousness, vomiting with skull changes of tense fontanellae, sun-setting eyes and increased skull diameter.

Chronic onset in adults tends to cause headache, nausea, vomiting and difficulty in upward gazing. When the hydrocephalus develops acutely, patients may demonstrate dementia, ataxia or incontinence.

Treatment

Endoscopic ventriculostomy may be effective in non-communicating hydrocephalus and has the advantage of leaving the patient shunt free. Ventricular shunting, the diversion of CSF from ventricles using subcutaneous shunt tubing to deliver the CSF to the peritoneal space, pleural space or the right atrium, is used in communicating hydrocephalus (Figure 7.5).

Figure 7.5 Coronal section of the ventricular system

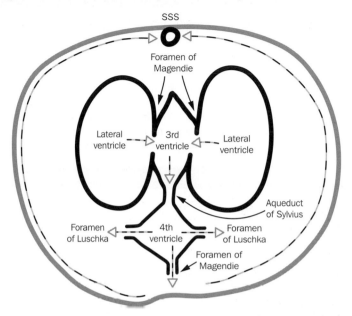

VENTRICULAR SHUNT PROBLEMS

Patients with shunts are always at risk of two serious complications: blockage and infection.

History

- Depressed consciousness level
- Fever
- Headache
- Nausea/vomiting or seizures

Examination

There may be pus/erythema over the shunt tract. The patient should be examined for signs of raised intracranial pressure.

Investigations

- CT scan
- MSU/sputum/blood cultures
- Electrolytes
- Levels of antiepileptics

Treatment

If a shunt complication is suspected, the patient must be referred to a neurosurgical unit. If previous scans are available (to compare with current ventricular size), and the results of the above investigations are to hand, these will be helpful when referring the patient.

INFECTIONS

EPIDURAL ABSCESS

History

Early stages of presentation are non-specific. This phase is followed by severe pain, at the site of the abscess. Systemic upset may be a feature followed by rapidly ensuing organ failure if left untreated. The most pointed feature is progressive loss of motor and sensory function, including loss of sphincter control. Respiratory compromise is a feature of high cervical lesions.

Investigations

Exquisite spinal tenderness on percussion is pathognomonic of epidural abscess. MRI with and without contrast (or CT if MRI unavailable).

Treatment

Urgent referral to a neurosurgical unit is indicated.

INTRACEREBRAL ABSCESS

The major differential diagnosis is glioblastoma. The lesion wall tends to be thick and irregular in the case of a glioblastoma. A lesion that is thin walled and regularly enhancing on CT suggests an abscess.

History

Suspicion may be aroused by a pre-existing systemic infection or sinusitis or mastoiditis, but systemic upset is often absent. Once suspected or diagnosed, urgent neurosurgical referral is indicated.

Examination

Present with focal deficit, decreased GCS or seizures.

Investigations

The appropriate investigation for diagnosis of an abscess is CT brain with and without contrast. The infection is usually mixed in aetiology.

Treatment

The most important treatment is often surgical, but antibiotics should be broad-spectrum, including Gram +ve, −ve and anaerobic cover.

Brainstem death and organ donation are dealt in Chapter 10

CHAPTER 8

PLASTIC SURGERY

N KHWAJA AND K DUNN

GRAFTS AND FLAPS

A graft is a free transfer of tissue without its own blood supply. Its survival is dependent on the recipient area having a good blood supply. Grafts usually consist of skin or bone but can also be cartilage or fat.

SKIN GRAFTS

Three types:

- Autograft – graft from one individual transferred to a different area on the same individual
- Allograft (homograft) – taken from another individual of same species
- Xenograft (heterograft) – taken from a different species

Grafts are subclassified depending on the thickness of the dermis taken. Skin grafts are either split thickness (SSG) or full thickness (FTSG). SSG consists of epidermis and a variable amount of dermis, which determines its thickness. FTSG includes all the dermis in addition to epidermis.

Skin grafts 'take' by:

- Adherence – fibrin bonds easily disrupted by shear forces and infection
- Plasmatic imbibition – graft swelling and oedema; contributes to nutrition
- Revascularisation – circulation restored in 4–7 days (thicker grafts take longer)

CAUSES OF SKIN GRAFT FAILURE

- Shear forces
- Haematoma
- Infection
- Unsuitable bed (avascular)

A flap is a unit of tissue that maintains its blood supply while being transferred from donor to recipient site. Flaps can be classified by (Table 8.1):

- Type of blood supply (random/pedicled)
- Technique of transfer (advancement/rotation/transposition/distant/free)
- Tissues incorporated in the flap (cutaneous/fasciocutaneous/musculocutaneous/muscle only)

Table 8.1 Examples of common flaps

Latissimus dorsi	Pedicle flap	Chest wall Breast Shoulder Neck
	Free flap	Scalp Head and neck Lower limb
Rectus abdominis TRAM (transverse rectus abdominis muscle) VRAM (vertical rectus abdominis muscle)	Pedicle flap	Breast Perineum
	Free flap	Upper and lower limbs Breast
Radial forearm flap	Pedicle flap	Hand
	Free flap	Head and neck Lower limb
Deep inferior epigastric artery perforator flap (DIEP)	Free flap	Breast
Gracilis	Pedicle flap	Perineum
	Free flap	Facial reanimation

Flap monitoring

It is essential to monitor the vascularity of flaps postoperatively, especially of free flaps (see Table 8.2 for causes of free flap failure), for prevention and early recognition and treatment of complications.

Assess:

- Colour
- Refill
- Temperature
- Bleeding on pinprick
- Doppler pulse

Table 8.2 Causes of free flap failure

Mechanical	Anastomosis problem Pedicle problem (kinked, twisted, stretched, compressed)
Hydrostatic	Inadequate perfusion Inadequate venous drainage
Thrombogenic	Vessels in zone of injury Traumatic pedicle dissection Hypercoagulable state Ischaemia-reperfusion injury

BURNS

In the UK, 0.5–1% of the population sustains burn each year. Of these, 10% require admission, of which 10% are life-threatening. In children, scalding is most common whereas in adults flame burns account for most injuries.

MECHANISMS OF BURNS

- Scald
- Flame
- Contact (eg iron)
- Electrical
- Chemical – acid/alkali/dyes/fertilisers
- Frostbite

History

It is essential to take a full detailed history particularly of the event(s) leading to the injury. If possible, speak to fire officers who were at the scene.

- Location – indoors/outdoors/vehicle/RTS (road traffic accident)
- Mechanism – water/flame/contact. Eg, if cup of tea – when it was made, was milk added (to estimate temperature of fluid)
- Clothes worn at time of incident
- First aid measures taken – were clothes removed/cooling (risk of hypothermia)
- Anyone else involved, eg road traffic accident/house fire
- Exact time of injury (for major burns)

If children involved, consider non-accidental injury (NAI), particularly if:

- Multiple injuries at different times
- Changing story – important to retake history

Examination

Surface area of the burn

Wallace's rule of 9s – provides an approximation of the area of skin burnt for adults (does not apply to children). The body is split up into units of surface area divisible by 9 (except the perineum). Usually, charts of area are available in most burns units. Lund and Browder charts – adult and paediatric charts – are available in most emergency departments. The surface area of the burn is evaluated on the basis that the **patient's** palm is approximately 1% of their total body surface area (more accurately 0.8%).

Table 8.3 Assessment of percentage burn area: the rule of 9s

Area	% Body surface area
Head	9
Anterior torso	18
Posterior torso	18
Each leg	18
Each arm	9
Genitalia/perineum	1

Note: when assessing the total body surface area of a burn do not include erythema.

Figure 8.1 Lund and Browder chart

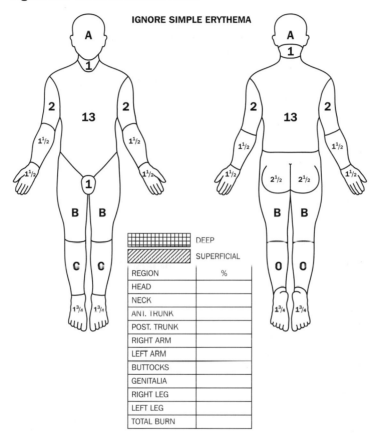

IGNORE SIMPLE ERYTHEMA

REGION	%
HEAD	
NECK	
ANT. TRUNK	
POST. TRUNK	
RIGHT ARM	
LEFT ARM	
BUTTOCKS	
GENITALIA	
RIGHT LEG	
LEFT LEG	
TOTAL BURN	

DEEP
SUPERFICIAL

RELATIVE PERCENTAGE OF BODY SURFACE AREA AFFECTED BY GROWTH

	Age (years)					
AREA	0	1	5	10	15	ADULT
A = $\frac{1}{2}$ of head	9.5	8.5	6.5	5.5	4.5	3.5
B = $\frac{1}{2}$ of one thigh	2.75	3.25	4	4.25	4.5	4.75
C = $\frac{1}{2}$ of one leg	2.5	2.5	2.75	3	3.25	3.5

Depth of burn

This is determined clinically by the appearance of the burn wound (see Table 8.4).

● Note any special areas involved (eg face/perineum)
● Signs of inhalation injury (see below) – carbonaceous sputum/hoarse voice/enclosed space fire

Table 8.4 Depth of burn as determined by appearance

Depth	Colour	Capillary refill	Sensation	Blisters	Healing
Superficial	Red	+	+	–	+
Superficial dermal	Pale pink	+	+	Small	+
Mid-dermal	Dark pink	Slow	+	Large	Usually
Deep dermal	Fixed staining	–	–	–	–
Full thickness	White/yellow	–	–	–	–

MINOR BURNS

Most burns do not require admission and many do not require specialised follow-up (see below). Ask for advice if in doubt whether a burn referral should be accepted (as inpatient or outpatient). Those injuries not needing admission may need following up in the burns or dressing clinic.

CRITERIA FOR BURNS UNIT REFERRAL

■ Burns at extremes of age (unless minor)
■ Burns > 5% total body surface area in children and > 10% in adults
■ Full thickness burn > 5% total body surface area in adults
■ Inhalation injury
■ Burns of special areas – face, perineum, hands/feet
■ Electrical or chemical burns
■ Burns requiring escharotomy
■ Any burns with suspicion of NAI
■ Burn associated with major trauma
■ Burns in patients with significant pre-existing illness

RESUSCITATION OF MAJOR BURNS

These patients may directly come to your hospital A&E or be transferred from another hospital local to where the incident occurred. The resuscitation discussed below is also useful as an aide memoire for referrals from other hospitals as they deal with these injuries infrequently.

A major burn requires a number of people to be ready in A&E. If you get a call alerting you to a patient with burns go to A&E to receive the patient as soon as they arrive. Ensure that a team is ready. Do not try to deal with the patient on your own with a nurse.

Try to get some basic history from the A&E staff. Often an anaesthetist will be needed from the outset. Make sure the following are available immediately:

- Fluids (Hartmann's) ideally warmed
- Intravenous cannulae (large bore)
- Blankets (to avoid hypothermia)
- Urinary catheter
- Equipment for intubation
- Burns charts – it is very useful to draw on the chart as you assess each part of the body

First aid at the scene
- Ensure safety of the rescuer
- Extinguish flames
- Remove burnt/soaked clothing – avoid hypothermia
- Switch off power source
- Cool the burn wound – this reduces direct thermal trauma and is analgesic
- Remove any residual burnt clothing
- Tepid water (does not have to be ice cold)
- Ambulance crews may use hydrocolloid gels at the scene
- Dilute acids and alkalis (see below)

On arrival in A&E
Approach patient as for any multiple trauma using ATLS principles.

Airway with cervical spine control and oxygen

- 100% high-flow oxygen
- Ensure an anaesthetist is present as the patient may need early intubation before swelling makes this difficult (facial burns, inhalation injury)

Breathing

- Assess for inhalation injuries
- The need for emergency chest escharotomy before senior help arrives is uncommon but assess any burns on the chest

Circulation with haemorrhage control and iv access

- Two large-bore cannulae preferably through non-burnt skin
- Avoid central venous cannulation in the initial stages
- Take blood for FBC, U&E, LFT, glucose, group and save or crossmatch, carboxyhaemoglobin and ABG
- Start fluid infusion 2 litres Hartmann's stat
- Urinary catheter

Disability – remembered by 'AVPU'. Classify patient's consciousness status as one of:

- **A**lert
- Respond to **V**oice
- Respond to **P**ain
- **U**nresponsive

Exposure

- Remove all clothing and jewellery
- Cover to keep warm
- Estimate total body surface area burnt using rule of 9s or a Lund and Browder chart
- Log roll to assess back
- Estimate depth (show by different shading on burn chart)
- Assess presence of full thickness circumferential limb burns (need for escharotomy)

Fluids – see below.

Secondary survey

- Head to toe examination
- Assess extent of burn injury
- Concomitant resucitation

FLUIDS

There are a number of formulae for fluid resuscitation of major burns – different for adults and children. Most use Parkland's formula. Another formula often used, especially for children, is Muir and Barclay's formula. **Check the protocols in your unit**.

Parkland's formula

To calculate fluid requirement: 4 ml × body weight (kg) × % total body surface burnt = fluid requirement in 24 hours.

- Give half in the first 8 hours **from the time of injury**
- Give the remaining half over the next 16 hours
- Children require maintenance fluid **in addition** to resuscitation fluid
- Use dextrose saline
- Watch for hypoglycaemia and hyponatraemia
- Monitoring fluid resuscitation with clinical parameters:

  ○ Pulse
  ○ Respiratory rate
  ○ Urine output 0.5 ml/kg adult or 1ml/kg children
  ○ Capillary refill

Note: Fluid formulae are guides only – patient must be monitored and reassessed.

INHALATION INJURY

Eighty per cent of fire-related deaths are due to inhalation injury. Always examine for inhalation injury as this affects management in A&E, transfer and long-term management. Above the larynx, heat causes thermal injury to upper airways. Below the level of the larynx, chemical injury is caused to the alveoli due to the dissolved acidic products of combustion. If inhalation injury is suspected, ITU assessment is needed for elective intubation as maximum upper airway oedema and narrowing occur approximately 24 hours after the injury.

Examination

- Look for facial burns and soot in mouth/nose
- **Hoarse voice/stridor**
- Dyspnoea
- Wheeze
- Tachypnoea
- Tachycardia
- Altered consciousness level
- Systemic examination – toxic effects of inhaled poisons

Investigations

- ABG
- Carboxyhaemoglobin
- CXR
- Fibreoptic bronchoscopy

Treatment

Intubation – this is much more difficult once the airway starts to become oedematous.

PAEDIATRIC BURNS

Many aspects of treatment are the same as for adults, but there are some important differences when treating children with burn injuries:

- Larger surface area:volume area ratio
- Higher circulating volume (80 ml/kg; adults – 60 ml/kg)
- Larger head, smaller lower limbs – need to adjust the rule of 9s
- Need to maintain a higher urine output (1–2 ml/kg per hour)
- Susceptible to hypoglycaemia and hyponatraemia
- Fluids can be administered by intraosseous route (under 6 years)
- Prone to hypothermia
- To assess the total body surface area involved use either the palm of the child's hand as 1% or a Lund and Browder chart
- Require maintenance fluid (dextrose saline) in addition to resuscitation fluid (Hartmann's solution):

  - Resuscitation fluid – as for adults: 4 ml $\times$ body weight (kg) $\times$ % body surface area burnt = ml over 24 hours
  - Half in the first 8 hours and half in the next 16 hours
  - Maintenance fluids 4 ml/kg per hour for the first 10 kg, adding 2 ml/kg per hour for the second 10 kg and 1 ml/kg per hour for each kg over 20 kg

OTHER BURNS

Electrical burns

Electrical burns classified as:

- Low voltage (<1000 Hz)

  - ○ Household voltage 240 V in UK
  - ○ Local tissue necrosis, cardiac symptoms, arrest

- High voltage (>1000 Hz)

  - ○ Muscle injury, compartment syndrome, myoglobinuria, cardiac symptoms

- Lightening strike

  - ○ Direct strike/side flash → cardiac arrest, compartment syndrome

Chemical burns

These continue to cause tissue damage after exposure. Determine exact nature of chemical, duration and site of exposure. Determine the type of chemicals involved: acids, alkali or other.

Acids

- Cause coagulative necrosis
- Irrigate with water
- Hydrofluoric acid – 10% calcium gluconate and copious irrigation with water, wound debridement

Alkali

- Liquefactive necrosis and severe pain
- Household bleaches, oven cleaners, fertilisers, cement
- Ocular injury – corneal scarring and ulceration
- Cement – dessication injury, delayed symptoms and presentation
- Phenol – copious water irrigation
- Bitumen/tar – cool burn wound (bitumen hardens)
- Paraffin dressings – absorb adherent bitumen
- Phosphorus – fertilisers/fireworks/insecticides/firearms
- Irrigation with water
- Monitor ECG
- Cardiac/renal/hepatic effects

BURN SURGERY

Immediate

- Excision
- Wound cover
- Escharotomy

Early

- Excision (tangential or fascial)
- Wound cover (skin graft/skin substitutes)

Late

- Post-burn reconstruction

HAND TRAUMA

Hand trauma forms the bulk of acute referrals to plastic surgery and most will require surgical treatment either under general or regional anaesthesia. Check your unit policy regarding accepting and treating referrals.

TYPES OF HAND INJURY

- Infection
- Burn
- Laceration
- Closed injury
- Fractures
- Bites
- Crush
- Degloving
- Finger tip injury
- Amputation
- Devascularisation

The following injuries should be seen as soon as referred:

- Infections
- Bites (where possible)
- Open fractures (where possible)
- Crush injuries
- Devascularisation of digit/hand/limb
- Amputation where replantation is considered (see below)

Less serious injuries (eg simple lacerations, tendon injury, finger tip injury) may be seen the following day. Check departmental policy and ensure:

- Prophylactic antibiotics
- Adequate analgesia
- Dressings – non-adherent and antiseptic
- Elevation – broad arm sling
- Splint (to help with pain relief)
- Instructions for starvation prior to surgery

When consenting for surgery for hand injuries remember to explain specifically:

- The resulting scars may be more extensive than the original injury
- Risk of infection (may need postoperative antibiotics)
- May have altered sensation/numbness postoperatively (local anaesthesia)
- Need for splint postoperatively (eg 6 weeks in tendon injuries)
- Importance of postoperative physiotherapy and occupational therapy
- Advice about driving/work

Assessment

Use the 'ABC' ATLS protocol for polytrauma. Limb injuries come under secondary survey BUT occasionally may come under 'C' as haemorrhage control.

History

Always remember to check for any other associated injuries depending on mechanism of injury (eg assaults, road traffic accident).

Also ask:

- Age
- Occupation
- Hobbies
- Hand dominance
- Previous hand injuries
- Mechanism of injury (laceration/crush/avulsion, etc)
- Time of injury
- Past medical history including smoking history, diabetes
- Tetanus status

Examination (always examine both hands)

- Look – perfusion, old scars, swellings, wasting, hand arcade, zone of injury
- Feel – sensation especially distal to injury, tender mass in palm
- Move – passive and active movements distal to injury
- Neurological examination of ulnar, median and radial nerves

Investigations

- FBC and crossmatch if bleeding
- X-ray: fractures/glass injuries/foreign bodies

Treatment

- Dressing – non-adherent indamine/Jelonet/Mepitel $\pm$ Betadine gauze
- Wool and crepe
- Splintage volar slab – hand in position of function
- Elevation
- Antibiotics
- Tetanus status
- Arrange for admission and theatre
- **Remember to remove rings from injured hand**

FLEXOR TENDON INJURIES

These are described by Verdan's zones (Figure 8.2).

Examination

Examine both hands.

Figure 8.2 Verdan's zones – flexor tendon injury

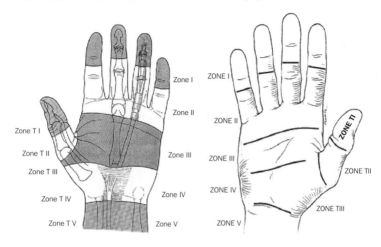

Remember when examining a hand for tendon injury:

- 15% do not have flexor digitorum superficialis (FDS) to little finger
- 15% have non-functioning FDS to ring and little finger
- Some have adhesions between FDS to little and ring fingers preventing independent movement

Linburg's sign:

- Flexor pollicis longus (FPL) action accompanied by flexion at distal interphalangeal (DIP) joint of index finger due to adhesions of FPL and FDP index in carpal tunnel

Treatment

All need examination under anaesthesia and tendon repair. It is useful to know where the end of the tendon is, to inform if significant wound extension of palm incision is required. Zone I repair may require re-insertion technique (button, screw). Re-do repairs can be difficult to manage and are often best dealt with semi-electively.

Keep NIL BY MOUTH 6 hours. Some units may use regional anaesthesia (not local).

Verdan's zones (Figure 8.3)

Figure 8.3 Verdan's zones – extensor tendon injury

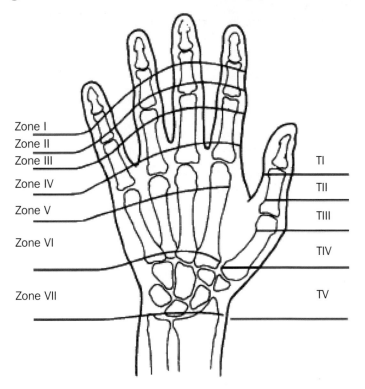

Zone I
Zone II
Zone III
Zone IV
Zone V
Zone VI
Zone VII

TI
TII
TIII
TIV
TV

MALLET FINGER

History

Forced flexion of extended digit.

Examination

- Open/closed
- Zone of poor vascularity at site of mallet ruptures

Table 8.5 Green's classification for mallet finger injury

Type I	Closed ± small avulsion fracture (most common)
Type II	Open
Type III	Open, loss of tendon
Type IV	A – transepiphyseal plate fracture B – fracture involving 20–50% articular surface (hyperflexion) C – hyperextension injury > 50% articular surface, volar subluxation

Treatment

- Type I stack splint 6 weeks
- Type II–IV surgical repair

FINGER TIP INJURIES

CAUSES

- Crush
- Laceration
- Blast

Table 8.6 Classification of finger tip injuries (Allen)

I	Skin and pulp distal to nail bed
II	Pulp and nail bed distal to bone
III	Loss of part of terminal phalanx
IV	Amputation proximal to nail bed

CHILDREN

- Usually nail bed lacerations, eg after finger caught in door
- Assess vascularity
- Most require nail bed repair under GA
- Some very distal injuries can be treated conservatively with dressings

Treatment options:

- Conservative
- Terminalisation
- Split-skin graft
- Composite graft
- Homodigital flap (flap from same finger as injury)
- Cross-finger flap (flap from adjacent finger)

REPLANTATION

Replantation/revascularisation involves long surgery and recovery with variable outcomes. Some patients will benefit from terminalisation as a primary procedure.

Below are some general principles and early management options prior to the decision for surgery being made. In addition to ATLS resuscitation and generic management of hand injury:

History

- Time of injury, ischaemia time
- Storage of amputated part – damp (not soaked) saline gauze within a plastic bag on ice

Examination

- Examination of amputated part
- Level of injury
- Extent of crush/avulsion
- Concomitant injuries

Investigations

X-ray of hand and amputated part.

See Table 8.7 for indications and contraindications to limb replantation.

Table 8.7 Limb replantation – indications and contraindications

Indications	Child
	Thumb amputation
	Multiple digits, whole hand/limb
Relative contraindications	Single digit amputation
	Avulsion of tendons, nerves, vessels
	Significant contamination
	Long warm ischaemia time
	Unwilling or uncooperative patient
Absolute contraindications	Head/thoraco-abdominal life-threatening injuries
	Multi-level injury, extensive crush or degloving
	Severe chronic illness

POSTOPERATIVE CARE

Principles similar to free flap surgery:

- Keep patient warm (ideally in a side room)
- Maintain good fluid balance (UO (urine output) > 1–2 ml/kg per hour)
- Analgesia
- Elevation – on pillows
- **Must** avoid smoking in the early postoperative period

White finger postoperatively (inflow problem)

- Ensure patient is warm, well filled and pain free (prevent hypoperfusion and spasm)
- Loosen dressings
- Remove sutures
- May need re-exploration

Blue finger postoperatively (outflow problem)

- Elevate limb
- Loosen dressings
- Remove sutures
- Leeches
- Anticoagulation
- May need re-exploration

Check with senior before removing dressings, sutures, etc.

MAJOR LIMB REPLANTATION

Patients who have had major limb replantation, such as a forearm, are at risk from reperfusion injury due to the muscle mass of the limb (see Chapter 3, Compartment syndrome, pages 131–133).

- Monitor – hyperkalaemia
- Renal function
- Myoglobinuria
- May need fasciotomy

HAND INFECTIONS

FINGERS

- Paronychial infection:

  - Commonest hand infection
  - *Staphylococcal aureus*

- Felon – abscess of pulp space
- Herpetic whitlow:

  - Herpes simplex virus vesicular eruption in the fingertip
  - Incision and drainage if secondary bacterial abscess

- Collar stud abscess – infection in subfascial palmar space pointing dorsally
- Flexor sheath infection:

  - Usually occur as result of penetrating injury to flexor sheath
  - Kanavel's four signs – sausage-shaped fusiform swelling; stiffness in semiflexed position; tenderness along flexor sheath into the palm; pain with passive extension
  - Requires drainage and irrigation of flexor sheath

PALMS

The palm has three potential spaces deep to the flexor tendons where an abscess may form. These will need surgical drainage.

Thenar space
- Lies radial to the oblique septum which extends downwards from the palmar fascia to the third metacarpal
- Flexor sheath infections of index finger may rupture into this potential space

Mid-palmar space
- Ulnar side of oblique septum
- Flexor sheath infections of middle and ring fingers may rupture into this space

Hypothenar space
- Rarely involved in hand infections

DORSAL HAND

There are two spaces in the dorsum of the hand where abscess may form.

Dorsal subcutaneous space
- Large space overlying the entire dorsum of hand
- Communicates in finger webs with potential space beneath palmar fascia and so palmar infections may spread to dorsum

Dorsal subaponeurotic space
- Just below extensor retinaculum

BITES

Organisms:

- Human bites – *Staphylococcus*, *Streptobacillus*, anaerobes
- Dog bites – *Pasteurella multocida*, *Streptobacillus*, *Staphylococcus*, anaerobes
- Cat bites – *Pasteurella multocida*

Bite injuries should generally be debrided/repaired within 6 hours of injury. Start on iv antibiotics early.

GENERAL PRINCIPLES

Both open and closed fractures of the hand are dealt with by plastic/hand surgeons but individual units will have their own protocols. In general:

- Open or closed fractures distal to the wrist (open or closed injury) are dealt with by plastic surgery
- Fractures proximal to the wrist are dealt with by orthopaedic surgery unless there is associated skin, soft tissue, tendon or neurovascular injury

Closed fractures can be treated by:

- Conservative treatment
- Manipulation under anaesthesia + fixation
- K-wire
- Open reduction and internal fixation (ORIF)

Unacceptable phalangeal fractures requiring surgical intervention include those with:

- Rotation
- Severe dorsal angulation
- Lateral angulation.
- Phalangeal fractures

Thumb fractures:

- Bennett's fracture – oblique fracture of the first metacarpal base is treated with traction on abductor pollicis longus tendon but usually requires ORIF
- Reversed Bennett's – is a similar fracture of the fifth metacarpal base and is treated with traction on extensor carpi ulnaris tendon
- Rolando fracture – is similar to Bennett's but with the avulsed segment a T-shape condylar fracture; needs ORIF

Table 8.8 Assessment of nerve injury

Motor	Median nerve	Abductor pollicis longus
	Ulnar nerve	Adductor digiti minimi/finger adduction
	Radial nerve	Finger extension
Sensory	Median nerve	Thenar eminence
	Ulnar nerve	Volar aspect little finger
	Dorsal branch of ulnar nerve	Dorsal aspect little finger
	Superficial radial nerve	Skin over anatomical snuff box

LOWER LIMB TRAUMA

Lower limb injuries may require plastic surgery referral for extensive soft-tissue injury requiring reconstruction.

COMPOUND FRACTURES

Described by Gustillo Anderson classification (Table 8.9).

History

- Mechanism of injury
- Full history of accident (guide to energy levels)
- High energy suggested by:
  - Road traffic accidents
  - Fall from significant height
  - Missile wounds
  - Crush injury

Examination

- High energy suggested by:
  - Large soft-tissue defect
  - Closed degloving injury
  - Presence of associated injuries
  - Segmental injuries
  - Imprints from dirt or tyres
  - Comminution of bony fragments

Table 8.9 Gustillo–Anderson classification of compound fractures

Grade I	Clean puncture wound Minimal muscle contusion No crush injury Simple fracture, no comminution
Grade II	Laceration > 1 cm diameter No extensive soft-tissue damage, flaps or avulsions Simple fracture, no comminution
Grade III	Extensive soft-tissue damage (skin, muscle and neurovascular structures) High energy and severe crushing component Comminuted fractures Segmental fracture Bone loss Gunshot wounds
Grade IIIa	High energy trauma regardless of wound size Adequate soft-tissue cover of bone
Grade IIIb	Extensive soft-tissue injury, periosteal stripping with bone exposure Major wound contamination Bone loss
Grade IIIc	Open fracture with arterial injury requiring repair

Treatment

- Fasciotomy – important not to jeopardise any future flaps
- Early surgical management:
    - Wound extension
    - Wound excision
    - Debridement of necrotic tissue
    - Lavage
    - Fracture stabilisation
- Soft-tissue cover – local or free flap

CHAPTER 9

EAR, NOSE AND THROAT

S KHWAJA AND S SAEED

In ENT it is essential to carry out a detailed head and neck examination, which in many cases will reveal the diagnosis without the need for investigation. Most A&E departments and ENT wards will have a supply of auriscopes, nasal speculum, head torches, etc, to allow complete examination. In many cases direct or indirect scopes or even fibreoptic endoscopes will be needed.

ENT EXAMINATION

EAR EXAMINATION

Look at the pinna from behind and in front and always compare your findings with the contralateral side. Look for operation scars, haematomas, cellulitis, perichondritis, discharge at the external auditory meatus (EAM) and cysts in the ear lobe. If there is ear pain examine the ear, pinna and behind the ear (mastoid). Pain may also be referred pain due to a nose, temporomandibular joint, teeth, throat or even the cervical spine cause.

To examine the ear canal use the otoscope with the correct-sized speculum and retract the pinna backwards for children and backwards and superiorly for adults. The entire external ear should be examined for swelling, erythema and discharge. It is also essential to ascertain if the eardrum is visible and if so describe the findings in terms of the four quadrants.

Weber's test is carried out using a 512-Hz tuning fork, which is held against the forehead in the midline, and asking the patient where the sound is heard. When both ears are normal there is either no localisation of sound or it is central. If there is a conductive hearing loss in one ear the patient will point to that ear. If there is a severe or profound sensorineural hearing loss in one ear the patient will point to the opposite ear.

Rinne's test involves placing the base of the 512-Hz tuning fork against the mastoid bone behind the ear and then in front of the EAM. The patient is asked to compare the sound heard from these two positions and to say which is louder. In a normal ear the air conduction is louder than the bone conduction or Rinne positive. If there is a conductive hearing loss, bone conduction (tuning fork held at the mastoid tip) is better than air conduction (tuning fork at the

EAM). This is because sound is transmitted directly to the cochlea through the bone while the sound travelling through the EAM is impaired or Rinne negative. If one ear has sensorineural hearing loss, sound will travel via bone conduction to the intact cochlea on the opposite side, described as Rinne-false-negative.

NOSE EXAMINATION

Examine the bridge of the nose and tip. Occlude each nostril separately to assess nasal airflow or use a metal spatula and assess nasal misting on expiration of nasal airflow. Anterior rhinoscopy is carried out using a Thudicum speculum and headlight to assess the septum for deviation, septal perforation, septal abscess, septal haematoma and bleeding points. Assess the nasal lining to see if it is wet and boggy or dry. Compare the nasal turbinates on each side and note any nasal polyps present. Assess the nasal cavity for nasal discharge, and if unilateral check if there is a foreign body or lesion present. If experienced in using Hopkins' rod, the post-nasal space should be examined or the patient should be assessed in a clinic where a senior can assess the post-nasal space.

THROAT EXAMINATION

You should always carry a pen, torch and tongue depressor with you. In a perfect world all wards should have a working otoscope with disposable ear pieces (speculums). Other useful equipment includes a tuning fork and nasendoscope, which should be available on an ENT ward. Always use two wooden or metal spatulas to carry out a thorough inspection of the oral cavity. Examine the teeth, buccal mucosa, tongue and palatal arches, tonsils if present and soft and hard palate and posterior oropharyngeal wall. Finally always palpate – with a gloved finger – the tongue, feeling for asymmetry or lesions. Examine the floor of mouth including balloting the submandibular glands. Assessment of the larynx is probably best left to a senior and requires the use of fibreoptic nasendoscopy and indirect laryngoscopy.

NECK EXAMINATION

Inspect the neck from behind and in front for asymmetry and signs of previous surgery or radiotherapy. You should be able to divide the neck into anterior and posterior triangles and should know the structures which lie within these triangles.

On palpation you should be able to identify any abnormality and be able to give a differential diagnosis by remembering what structures lie in that area. Depending on your differential, other systems may need to be examined such as chest, axilla, groin and abdomen.

NEUROLOGICAL EXAMINATION

You should be proficient in assessing the cranial nerves and the peripheral nervous system.

Note: It is important to carry out a vocal cord check, before and after thyroid/parathyroid surgery.

PINNA HAEMATOMA

History

Pinna haematoma is usually secondary to trauma and is due to the collection of blood under the perichondrium.

Examination

Pinna haematomas tend to present with a fluctuant mass that is tender on palpation. If left untreated the cartilage may undergo necrosis with fibrous scarring, hence the characteristic 'cauliflower ear' of rugby players.

Treatment

The haematoma needs to be drained under aseptic conditions to prevent cartilage necrosis leading to permanent deformity. Aspiration with a needle and 5-ml syringe will confirm the diagnosis and drain small haematomas. Larger haematomas may need an incision and a Yates' drain under GA. A pressure dressing is required after the procedure to prevent re-collection. Antibiotic cover and analgesia should be provided and the patient reviewed in 2 days in outpatients. Make sure to check tetanus status and update as appropriate.

PINNA LACERATION

History

There is usually a history of trauma with or without contamination.

Examination

It is important to ascertain if the cartilage is also injured.

Treatment

Assess for cartilage loss and if there is enough skin to cover any exposed cartilage then primary closure should be performed under local anaesthesia after thorough cleansing using antiseptic solution. Antibiotic cover should be provided for a week and tetanus status should be checked. Stitches should be removed in 5 days and the patient reviewed in outpatients.

PERICHONDRITIS

History

Perichondritis is infection of the ear cartilage due to laceration of the pinna, following surgery or secondary to otitis externa. As with any abscess or unusual infection it is important to ascertain whether the patient is immunosuppressed or has diabetes.

Examination

If there is associated facial cellulitis, mark the extent of the infection to observe the spread of infection.

Treatment

When this is secondary to otitis externa it is important to treat the underlying condition with iv anti-staphylococcal and anti-staphyloccocal antibiotics. If the pinna is markedly oedematous, glycerol and ichthammol dressings can help decrease the swelling.

OTITIS EXTERNA

History

Patients tend to describe otalgia, with associated ear discharge and itchiness. There may also be hearing loss if the canal is swollen or purulent discharge occludes the canal. It is important to elicit a history of recent travel and swimming.

Examination

In addition to pain and discharge from the ear there may be associated facial cellulitis and pinna tenderness on movement.

Investigations

Send a swab for culture and sensitivity.

Treatment

Remove the discharge with swab brush and suction the ear using a microscope. If a microscope is not available, superficially clean the external auditory meatus. Assess the canal and if patent prescribe oral analgesia with topical antibiotics such as dexamethasone with antibacterial (Sofradex), gentamicin with hydrocortisone (Gentisone HC) drops or ciprofloxacin drops. Arrange a review in outpatients for 7 days but if the canal is oedematous, insert a pope wick with antibiotic cover and review in outpatients in 48 hours to assess for the need for suction clearance. You may also need to add oral ciprofloxacin. Admit patients with cellulitis or severe pain for iv antibiotics and analgesia. If there is a suggestion of resistant ear discharge or excessive ear itchiness or a confirmed swab result of a fungal infection, treat with 1% clotrimazole ear drops for at least 2 weeks.

EXTERNAL MEATUS/SKULL BASE OSTEITIS

History

External meatus/skull base osteitis is a rare condition, formerly known as 'malignant otitis externa', and seen in elderly, diabetic or immunocompromised patients. It involves inflammation and damage of the bones and cartilage of the base of the skull. It is caused by the spread of infection from an external ear infection with *Pseudomonas aeruginosa* or *Streptococcus milleri*.

Treatment

Admit for iv antibiotics and analgesia.

FURUNCLE

History

- Tender localised swelling in the external auditory meatus, usually caused by *Staphylococcus aureus* infection
- More common in immunocompromised or diabetic patients

Treatment

- These can be treated conservatively with magnesium sulphate dressings
- If the swelling is pointing it is worth carrying out an incision and drainage procedure followed by a course of anti-staphylococcal antibiotics

EAR FOREIGN BODY

History

There is usually a clear history, often with recurrent presentations.

Treatment

Remove the foreign object using a microscope if the ear drum is intact. Only remove if microscope, appropriately trained staff and instruments are available. However if the drum has been pierced or the patient (child) is uncooperative seek senior opinion.

EAR CANAL TUMOURS

History

These can be benign lesions such as exostoses and papilloma, or malignant lesions such as squamous cell carcinoma. They are often an incidental asymptomatic finding but occasionally present with discharge from the ear or intractable pain.

Investigations

Biopsy will provide histological diagnosis but it is important to have a CT scan to assess extent and to plan definitive treatment.

Treatment

If there is intractable pain it may be necessary to admit for analgesia. Surgery in the case of malignant disease can be complicated and may require the use of flaps to achieve adequate removal and closure.

TYMPANIC MEMBRANE PERFORATION

History

Commonly caused by direct trauma or as part of a head injury but may also result from barotrauma. Patients usually describe a bloody discharge and sudden loss of hearing.

Examination

Otoscopy will confirm the presence and location of the perforation and a CNS examination must be performed to record any associated injury especially to the facial (VII) nerve or vestibulocochlear (VIII) nerve.

Treatment

Usually these patients are admitted under another specialty for head injury observations. Tympanic membrane perforations rarely require immediate treatment and it is safe to keep the ear dry and provide analgesia until they can be reviewed in the outpatient clinic. However, if there is an associated facial nerve injury inform your senior who will advise on how to manage the case.

ACUTE OTITIS MEDIA

History

This typically presents with a systemic illness with fever and deep-seated ear pain associated with conductive deafness. If the drum perforates, the pain and fever will settle but there will be initial bloody then a purulent discharge. When the infection is slow to improve or associated with tenderness or swelling over the mastoid, unresolved acute otitis media should be suspected. This is a distinct condition where the patient is toxic with a prominent ear. There may also be an associated facial palsy, labyrinthitis, lateral sinus thrombophlebitis, extradural abscess, subdural abscess, brain abscess or even frank meningitis.

Examination

- Otoscopy to check whether perforation has occurred and the type of discharge associated
- If the condition fails to resolve a CT scan including temporal bones is necessary to rule out any of the above

Treatment

Oral analgesia, decongestants and antibiotics are usually sufficient to control simple otitis media with review by the patient's general practitioner in 1–2 weeks. Unresolved otitis media will require admission, iv antibiotics and possible surgical management depending on findings.

Note: Children may get recurrent acute otitis media. In this case swab the ear and treat with the appropriate antibiotic and refer to the paediatric ENT outpatients for assessment.

CHRONIC SUPPURATIVE OTITIS MEDIA

History

There is usually chronic history of discharging ear, no pain, but a decrease in hearing.

Treatment

Review in outpatients department for definitive treatment unless there are associated neurological signs, in which case admit and inform senior.

CHOLESTEATOMA

History

- Chronic history of smelly discharging ear
- No pain
- Decrease in hearing

Examination

Otoscopy may reveal squamous debris in the ear canal originating from the supero-posterior aspect of the ear drum or limited by ear discharge.

Treatment

Review in outpatients for definitive treatment unless there are associated neurological signs, in which case admit and inform senior.

CONDUCTIVE HEARING LOSS

CAUSES OF CONDUCTIVE HEARING LOSS

- Wax/foreign body
- Otitis media with effusion
- Ossicular chain discontinuity
- Otosclerosis

History

- It is important to ascertain any preceding history of recent upper respiratory tract infection or trauma
- Recent history of pregnancy should be recorded, as there is an association with otosclerosis

Examination

- Assess hearing using tuning fork
- Post nasal space needs to be examined to rule out other causes for the symptoms

Treatment

All patients should be reviewed in outpatients with formal assessment of hearing. If there is a recent history of an upper respiratory tract infection and the patient has fluid behind the tympanic membrane consider topical nasal decongestion, as this may improve the symptoms.

Note: In children, glue ear (otitis media with effusion) is a common cause for conductive hearing loss. These children should be referred to the ENT outpatients for further management.

SENSORINEURAL HEARING LOSS

Hearing loss can occur secondary to damage to the vestibulocochlear nerve directly or anywhere along the auditory pathway.

History

Causes for sensorineural hearing loss need to be assessed. It is important to differentiate between acquired causes and congenital deafness. So include questions about noise exposure, arterial disease, autoimmune conditions and history of ototoxic drugs.

Recent bacterial ear infection, viral infections (measles, mumps), sexually transmitted infection, or meningitis may indicate a post-infective cause. Unilateral deafness should bring up the possibility of vestibular schwannoma. Hearing loss can also be associated with a balance disorder such as Ménière's disease and peripheral vestibular upset. It is also important to exclude trauma as a cause.

Examination

- Tuning fork test will confirm sensorineural hearing loss
- ENT examination may be normal or point to the cause of the hearing loss
- Neurological examination is essential

Investigations

- Pure tone audiogram to confirm level of hearing loss and that it is sensorineural in origin
- MRI may be required to assess if there is a cerebellopontine angle lesion if hearing loss is unilateral

Treatment

Depends on cause of hearing loss – discuss with senior.

VERTIGO

History

- Hallucinations of movement, often associated with nausea or vomiting
- May be rotatory, swaying or falling
- Duration and in which position
- Any associated tinnitus or aural pressure

Examination

Need to assess cranial nerves and peripheral nervous system to rule out a vascular cause or cerebellar or cerebral lesion.

Investigations

MRI scan to rule out a central cause if symptoms do not improve.

Treatment

- Symptomatic relief – anti-emetics and rehydration
- Follow-up in outpatients to arrange further investigations if settled while in-patient

NASAL TRAUMA

History

There is usually a clear history of recent trauma.

Examination

Assess for associated facial, orbital (blow-out fracture) and head injury as well as the infraorbital nerve. It is important to note any septal haematoma or CSF rhinorrhoea.

Treatment

- If simple nasal fracture reassess in a week to decide if further management is required
- Facial or orbital fractures may require maxillofacial and ophthalmology input
- Septal haematoma or abscess needs incision and drainage under GA

EPISTAXIS

History

This is a common cause of referral from A&E. It is essential to record the side, precipitating event, duration of bleeding and any action taken to halt bleeding. Often there is a history of previous bleeds and admissions due to nosebleeds. Precipitating factors include the use of anticoagulants, bleeding diathesis, old age and hypertension.

Examination

Evaluate the volume of blood loss.

Investigations

- FBC
- Clotting
- Group and save

Treatment

It may be necessary to resuscitate the patient. If the bleeding is not brisk, assess if there is an anterior bleeding point, which can be cauterised under local anaesthesia and Otrivine (antazoline sulphate 0.5%, xylometazoline hydrochloride 0.05%), a rapidly acting vasoconstrictor. Cauterise using silver nitrate. If there is a brisk anterior bleed or a posterior bleed then 'pack' the nasal cavity in question and prescribe antibiotics.

Anterior bleeds can be packed with a Merocel pack or Rapid Rhino. Posterior bleeds can be controlled with a Rapid Rhino, but if this is unsuccessful a Brighton balloon, which has an anterior and posterior balloon, or a Foley catheter in the post-nasal space with a BIPP (bismuth iodine paraffin paste) pack anteriorly may be used. The Foley catheter's balloon is filled with water until it is visible in the oral cavity and then pulled forward until resistance is met. Secure it in position with an umbilical cord clamp but make sure the clamp is not pressing on the nasal tip or columella otherwise skin necrosis can occur. The patient will not tolerate this well and may require some anxiolytic. Make sure this is not excessive for the patient.

If bleeding continues prepare the patient for theatre.

Following treatment of the epistaxis, follow-up in outpatients is required for a formal examination of the nasal cavity and post-nasal space to rule out other causes for nose bleeds beside nasal vessels.

FOREIGN BODY IN THE NOSE

This is a common occurrence in children and can be challenging to deal with.

Treatment

Do not attempt to remove unless adequately trained staff and instruments are available. In the case of a battery or organic material it is worth considering emergency removal.

ACUTE SINUSITIS

History

This is characterised by facial pain, headaches or nasal congestion following an upper respiratory tract infection. This can be serious as if unresolved can lead to a periorbital cellulitis, diplopia and subperiosteal abscess formation.

Examination

It is important to illict any eye symptoms/signs such as red colour vision change, chemosis, proptosis or ophthalmoplegia, which may indicate more serious infection.

Investigations

Patients with any of the above indicators of more serious infection warrant urgent admission and a CT scan of the paranasal sinuses.

Treatment

- If simple sinusitis treat with alternating nasal decongestant drops and steroid nasal drops every 2 hours and oral antibiotics
- More serious cases will require admission and iv antibiotics

TONSILLITIS, GLANDULAR FEVER, QUINSY

History

- Patients present with sore throat, pyrexia, dysphagia and otalgia of varying duration
- If other people are unwell and there is associated cervical lymphadenopathy consider glandular fever
- If symptoms are unilateral and there is associated trismus consider a quinsy

Examination

- Oral examination for the size, shape and symmetry of any swelling around the palatine tonsil
- Trismus and a unilateral swelling around the tonsil pushing the tonsil and uvula to the opposite side are diagnostic for peritonsillar abscess (quinsy)

Investigations

- FBC
- Paul Bunnell test/Monospot to exclude infectious mononucleosis (glandular fever)

Treatment

Admit if clinically unwell for fluids and antibiotics. Monitor the airway especially for obstructive breathing which may require the patient to sleep upright initially. If Monospot is positive stop antibiotics unless there is a secondary bacterial infection and avoid penicillin-based antibiotics as these can lead to a rash. If there is little improvement consider a short course of iv/oral steroids.

Quinsy needs draining by aspiration or incision and the pus sent for culture and sensitivity.

POST-TONSILLECTOMY BLEEDS

History

Primary haemorrhage occurs during the surgery while reactionary haemorrhage occurs in the first 24 hours after surgery. Secondary haemorrhage occurs after 24 hours and up to 2 weeks postoperatively and is usually due to secondary infection of the tonsillar fossae.

Examination

Assess volume of blood loss and if there is active blood loss in the oral cavity.

Investigations

- FBC
- U&E
- Clotting
- Group and save

Treatment

- Establish iv access and commence iv fluids
- Keep the patient nil by mouth
- Consider hydrogen peroxide gargles
- For secondary haemorrhage commence appropriate iv antibiotics
- Inform senior early on

OESOPHAGEAL FOREIGN BODY

History

Ingestion of meat/foreign body followed by dysphagia. Drooling indicates absolute dysphagia. Time taken from a drink of water to regurgitating the water guides you to the level of obstruction.

Investigations

Soft-tissue lateral cervical spine X-ray and CXR. If not sure if there is a foreign body present or suspicion of underlying pathology request a contrast swallow to see if there is any obstruction.

Treatment

IM hyoscine butylbromide or diazepam can be tried if the foreign body did not contain bone or was not sharp. If the foreign body is in the distal oesophagus, ask the general surgeon to perform a flexible gastroscopy. If meat bolus contains bone or if the foreign body was sharp admit for iv fluids and start on iv cefuroxime and metronidazole and prepare the patient for theatre. If there is no bone or sharp objects it is not necessary to prescribe antibiotics. The patient can be observed overnight for the next day operating list. The patient should be observed for any signs of perforation (temperature, tachycardia, pain between the shoulder blades or central).

All patients need to be reviewed in outpatients following a contrast swallow result following this admission to rule out any underlying pathology.

STRIDOR AND STERTOR

Stridor is noisy breathing on inspiration because of upper airway obstruction usually at the level of the vocal cords or below in the trachea. See Table 9.1 for the possible causes. Stertor is characterised by noisy breathing due to a partial obstruction above the vocal cord level. See Table 9.2 for the possible causes.

History

Stridor and stertor can be associated with varying levels of respiratory distress. Treatment depends on the cause but the situation can deteriorate rapidly so it may be necessary to have an anaesthetist present. Always inform your senior early on.

Table 9.1 Causes of stridor

Congenital	Supraglottis	Laryngomalacia Web Saccular cyst Cystic hygroma
	Glottis	Web, vocal cord paralysis
	Subglottis	Web stenosis, haemangioma, cyst
	Trachea and bronchi	Web, stenosis, tracheomalacia, tracheo- and bronchogenic cysts External compression from mediastinal pathology
Acquired	Trauma	Thermal, chemical, iatrogenic, blunt and sharp
	Inflammatory/infective	Acute laryngitis, croup, subglottic cysts, vocal cord palsy
	Foreign body	
	Allergic	
	Neoplastic	Papillomas, laryngeal cancer, thyroid cancer

Examination

Do not examine the throat, especially if you suspect acute epiglottitis. Look at the patient at rest, assess tracheal tug, subcostal recession, nasal flaring and pulse oximetry. Look at the position of the patient to assess if accessory muscles of respiration are being used.

Investigations

No tests are required in the acute phase but if there was a diagnosis of angioneurotic oedema or an anaphylactic reaction consider testing for C1 esterase inhibitor titre.

Treatment

Monitor airway but do not examine patient using any instrumentation including a tongue depressor, endoscopy or direct laryngoscopy as this

Table 9.2 Causes of stertor

Congenital	Nose	Choanal stenosis Craniofacial abnormality Meningo/encephalocele Cysts
	Nasopharynx	Craniofacial abnormality Adenoidal hypertrophy
	Oropharynx	Micrognathia Macroglossia Lingual thyroid Thyroglossal cyst
Acquired	Trauma	Nasal/midfacial
	Inflammatory	Adenoiditis Acute tonsillitis Parapharyngeal abscess Retropharyngeal abscess Ludwig's angina Acute epiglottitis (HIB) Laryngo-reflux
	Foreign body	
	Allergy	Angioneurotic oedema of the floor of mouth
	Neoplasia – benign	Angiofibroma Nasal polyps
	Neoplasia – malignant	

can trigger a respiratory arrest. Wait for senior or anaesthetist to arrive to assess the airway. Sit the patient up and treat with high-flow oxygen (10–15 litres) delivered via a reservoir mask, humidified if possible. It may be required to use 3 ml of 1:1000 adrenaline nebulised in 2 ml of saline repeated as required every 30 minutes, and IV hydrocortisone 200 mg. See BNF.

Alternatives include Heliox – brown and white quartered cylinder (21% oxygen/79% helium). If respiratory distress continues intubation or a surgical airway may be required. It is also essential to treat the underlying infection with antibiotics. If the cause of stridor is trauma this may require surgical exploration. Add iv antihistamines to adrenaline and steroids if anaphylaxis is suspected. Consider iv hydrocortisone if there is an inflammatory cause.

If the patient has significant stertor and lowered consciousness level, consider a nasopharyngeal airway.

ADDITIONAL FEATURES TO CONSIDER IN CHILDREN

History

Ask about the duration of noisy breathing and if louder in certain positions, any abnormality in the crying or problems feeding and weight gain. A history of recent upper respiratory tract infection should be noted. It is important to elicit any past medical history including birth history, congenital abnormality and previous intubation/tracheostomy.

Examination

Do not examine the throat, especially if you suspect acute epiglottitis.

Look at the child at rest, assess tracheal tug, subcostal recession, nasal flaring and cyanosis. Ask mother to move the child in different positions. SaO_2 monitoring is useful.

Treatment

Provide oxygen, and if possible Heliox, to the child without causing distress. Use 400 mcg/kg (max 5 mg) of 1:1000 adrenaline nebulised in 3 ml of saline. See BNF. If there is a history of croup, a steroid nebulised can also be given. Inform senior early including anaesthetist. Depending on the degree of respiratory distress, the child might need a direct laryngotracheal bronchoscopy and intubation.

PENETRATING NECK INJURIES

History

Note history of implement causing the injury, time of injury and volume of blood loss.

Examination

Assess **A**irway, **B**reathing and **C**irculation. Record the point of penetration and if present the exit point of the implement.

Investigations

Depend on the resuscitation status of the patient.

Treatment

- Resuscitate the patient
- Exploration will be required in theatre
- If vascular injury, the vascular team will need to be informed

NECK SPACE INFECTIONS

History

Neck swelling associated with the patient being toxic. Usually caused by Ludwig's angina, a parapharyngeal abscess or a retropharyngeal abscess.

Examination

Assess the airway, if possible perform an ENT examination without distressing the patient.

Investigations

- FBC
- Blood film
- U&E
- Monospot
- Blood cultures – toxoplasmosis
- Tuberculosis
- Lateral soft-tissue neck X-ray and CXR
- Occasionally may need CT scan for deep-seated infections

Treatment

Protect the airway and commence patient on iv antibiotics, analgesia. May require surgical treatment. Inform senior of admission and your assessment of the airway.

This is a common condition characterised by acute lower motor neurone palsy. It is graded according to the House–Brackmann scale.

CAUSES OF FACIAL NERVE PALSY

- Viral as in herpes varicella; Ramsey–Hunt syndrome is a herpes zoster infection affecting the ear and occasionally the glossopharyngeal (IX) nerve
- Idiopathic, known as Bell's palsy
- Tumour
- Head trauma/facial trauma
- Ear infection – chronic suppurative otitis media, cholesteatoma, acute otitis media, malignant otitis externa
- Central causes – multiple sclerosis, gliomas, cerebrovascular accident, myasthenia gravis or Guillain–Barré syndrome
- Other causes – sarcoid, drugs

With any facial nerve lesion it is important to decide if this is the presentation of a tumour, eg cerebellopontine tumour, facial schwannoma, parotid tumour or squamous cell carcinoma of the ear canal. So MRI and/or CT scanning will be required.

Investigations and treatment of facial nerve palsy depend on the aetiology. Bell's palsy should be treated as a presumptive viral infection with aciclovir 800 mg five times a day for a week and adequate analgesia. A pope wick and antibiotic/steroid drops may be necessary if there is severe otalgia. Oral steroids are optional. Facial palsy associated with ear infection will require CT brain, and high definition temporal bone views in order to rule out associated temporal lobe abscess and to define the extent of infection, osteitis or cholesteatoma.

Note: If facial nerve was injured at the time of the head trauma/facial trauma it will need exploring urgently, otherwise observe for recovery. It is essential in this situation to assess hearing also. Central cause requires referral to a neurologist for investigation and treatment.

FACIAL CELLULITIS

History

Usually the patient presents with a spreading facial erythematous rash with associated oedema. The underlying cause may be eczema or an acute sinusitis.

Treatment

Admit the patient and treat with broad-spectrum iv antibiotics. If not treated effectively there is a risk of cavernous sinus thrombosis due to retrograde thrombophlebitis via the facial vein draining into the ophthalmic veins. Always look out for any eye symptoms or signs.

CHAPTER 10

CRITICAL CARE

M O MURPHY AND J GREENWOOD

It may seem obvious or second nature that patients who deteriorate and become seriously ill, either in the community or while an in-patient, are quickly recognised. However, this is not always the case. Deterioration may take many forms, from sudden cardiorespiratory arrest to subtle abnormalities in vital signs heralding impending crisis. The skill is to be able to recognise the latter before it becomes the former.

OBJECTIVE ASSESSMENT

Many hospitals have now introduced an early warning score (EWS) system in many ward areas (Table 10.1). Typically, acute admissions to hospital, postoperative patients and those in whom deterioration has been noted clinically have such a score measured.

Table 10.1 Modified early warning score system

	3	2	1	0	1	2	3
Heart rate (beats per minute)		< 40	41–50	51–100	101–110	111–129	> 130
Respiratory rate (breaths per minute)		< 9		9–14	15–20	21–29	> 30
Temperature (°C)		< 35		35–38.4		> 38.4	
Systolic blood pressure (mmHg)	< 70	71–80	81–100	101–199		> 199	
Conscious level (AVPU)				Alert	Reactive to VOICE	Reactive to PAIN	UN-RESPONSIVE

The system varies from hospital to hospital, but broadly consists of monitoring:

- Heart rate
- Respiratory rate
- Temperature
- Systolic blood pressure
- Consciousness level

Variation around a set of predefined normal ranges will attain a score, the total of which can help to identify a seriously ill patient.

A new score of 3 or more, or a deterioration of 2 or more obligates medical review within 30 minutes. If the score deteriorates by 1, many protocols allow a nursing intervention such as giving fluid or oxygen. When faced with a patient who is newly 'scoring' on their EWS, a quick clinical assessment should be followed by an arterial blood gas and discussion with a senior colleague.

The EWS is highly sensitive at identifying seriously ill patients, and has been shown to improve survival and decrease morbidity in areas in which it has been introduced. It may seem like a bit of a bind when constantly faced with calls regarding patients who are 'scoring', but it is vital to take this seriously and appreciate the importance of rapid review.

MONITORING

On the intensive care unit you will be faced with a bewildering array of monitoring screens, lines and tubes attached to all the patients. It can be difficult to know what all these measurements are used for, what they mean and how they are obtained. The following is a basic guide.

INVASIVE ARTERIAL BLOOD PRESSURE MONITORING

A fine-bore cannula placed in an artery, usually the radial or femoral, and is connected to a pressure transducer via a column of heparinised saline. It gives a constant, real-time reading of arterial blood pressure, as well as an access point for obtaining blood samples. Any patient on a ventilator or vasoactive drugs must have an arterial line in. Variation in the height of the arterial tracing is described as 'swing' on the arterial line and is a crude indicator of hydration status.

CENTRAL LINE AND MONITORING

A central line is a catheter which sits in a large central vein. It is usually inserted via the internal jugular or subclavian vein and the tip sits in the superior vena cava and can have three or four lumens. The distal port can be attached to a pressure transducer and is used to measure the central venous pressure (CVP). The other lumens are usually used to give drugs, especially vasopressors, which should only be given via a CVP line.

The CVP is useful as it gives a guide to the patient's fluid balance status. A typical value in a euvolaemic patient is 8–10 mmHg. The absolute value is of less importance than the trend. For example, a patient with a low CVP usually requires fluid, and when this is given the CVP will increase.

CONTINUOUS CARDIAC OUTPUT MONITORING

Continuous cardiac output monitoring (PiCCO) is a system for continuous and minimally invasive monitoring of cardiac output and other values. It consists of a special arterial catheter inserted in a central (usually femoral) artery, and a temperature-sensing injection port attached to the CVP line. The arterial line and guide wire are fragile, and may be difficult to insert in patients with peripheral vascular disease. By measuring temperature changes following the injection of ice-cold saline, it can work out the patient's cardiac output, systemic vascular resistance and other values which can help with the choice and dosing of inotropes and vasopressors. Other derived values such as intrathoracic blood volume can help with fluid balance.

PULMONARY ARTERY CATHETER

Following the introduction of PiCCO, the use of the pulmonary artery (PA) catheter has declined markedly. It is useful in patients in whom it is not possible to insert a PiCCO line, or in those where an accurate estimation of left heart filling pressure and PA pressure is required. The PA (Swan–Ganz) catheter is essentially a long CVP catheter with a balloon on the end. The inflated balloon is used to float the end of the catheter through the right side of the heart and the main pulmonary artery. It wedges in a small pulmonary artery and tamponades the circulation. Thus, the pressure at the tip of the catheter distal to the balloon (the wedge pressure) is approximately that of the left atrial filling pressure.

MECHANICAL VENTILATION

Many patients on the critical care unit will require mechanical ventilation at some stage to treat respiratory failure or protect the unconscious patient. There are numerous strategies, protocols and modes for artificially ventilating patients. In general, control of ventilation is either by pressure control, where the pressure of each breath is set to achieve the desired tidal volume, or volume control, where the desired tidal volume is set for each breath. In most cases volume control is used in conjunction with pressure regulation to ensure a set airway pressure is not exceeded. The following is a guide to the terminology and principles used.

SEDATED PATIENT

- **Continuous mandatory ventilation** (CMV): also known as intermittent positive pressure ventilation (IPPV). This mode uses a ventilator to deliver a set number of breaths per minute at a set pressure or volume (see below) in a patient who is making no intrinsic respiratory effort, ie they are paralysed or deeply unconscious.
- **Synchronised intermittent mandatory ventilation** (SIMV): this mode can function in the same way as CMV, in that it will deliver a set number of breaths at a set volume or pressure. However, if the patient initiates some of the breaths, the ventilator will sense this and augment, rather than oppose, the breath.
- **Spontaneous (pressure support) ventilatory support**: in this mode, the patient is breathing for themselves, initiating every breath, but the ventilator is delivering a pressure to the end of inspiration (the pressure support) and to the end of expiration (positive end-expiratory pressure, PEEP). Patients can be weaned in this mode.

AWAKE PATIENT

The above modes require a patient to have airway control, ie an endotracheal tube or tracheostomy. Ventilatory support can be delivered in an awake patient via a face mask. In this situation, the technique used can be CPAP or non-invasive ventilation (NIV).

CPAP is useful in patients with type I respiratory failure (eg pneumonia, pulmonary oedema). This delivers high-flow, high-concentration oxygen plus PEEP to each breath, thus increasing gas exchange. NIV is essentially pressure support ventilation via a face mask, and is useful for treating acute type II respiratory failure and in continuing weaning of the extubated patient. Weaning refers to the gradual reduction in ventilator support given to an improving patient. It requires there to be no active sepsis or thoracic pathology, an awake, co-operative, spontaneously breathing patient and compliance by the medical and nursing staff.

ACUTE RESPIRATORY DISTRESS SYNDROME

Acute respiratory distress syndrome (ARDS) is a syndrome of acute lung injury causing severe and often refractory respiratory failure. Often seen as a response to sepsis (see below), the basic pathological process is of increased capillary permeability in response to inflammatory mediators, causing a leakage of fluid into the extracellular space within the lungs. When occurring in enough of the lungs, this causes respiratory failure and makes the lungs 'stiff' and difficult to ventilate due to increased compliance.

The treatment of ARDS has been subject to much controversy in recent years. While treatment of the underlying cause is obviously needed, the role of high-dose steroids and various ventilatory strategies has now been discounted. The best evidence is currently for a lung-protective strategy employing low tidal volumes to avoid pressure-induced lung barotrauma. Tidal volumes of 6 ml per kg body weight should be used with a high PEEP.

In severe ARDS or respiratory failure refractory to standard ventilation, various strategies have been looked at. Many units will practise prone ventilation, or use a high-frequency oscillator ventilator. Both of these interventions may transiently improve oxygenation, but they do not have an influence on survival.

SEPSIS

Sepsis is the body's response to infection. Many patients admitted to the critical care unit have severe sepsis or septic shock. The mortality of septic shock despite full intensive care intervention is still up to 50%.

In sepsis, the initial insult is inflammation of some sort, most commonly due to a bacterial infection. The initial response is the systemic inflammatory response syndrome (SIRS). SIRS diagnosis requires the presence of two or more of:

- Heart rate > 90 beats per minute
- Respiratory rate > 20 breaths per minute or pCO_2 < 4.2 kPa
- Temperature > 38°C or < 36°C
- WCC >12 × 10^{-9}/l or < 4 × 10^{-9}/dl

Sepsis is defined as the presence of SIRS with an identified infection site. In some patients, the presence of SIRS leads to a massive circulation of inflammatory mediators. These mediators cause activation of the coagulation cascade, leaking of the capillaries and hypotension. The hypercoagulable state leads to microthrombosis in capillaries, disseminated intravascular coagulation, hypoperfusion and organ system dysfunction and failure.

The hallmark of severe sepsis seen on the critical care unit is hypotension and multiorgan failure:

- Respiratory failure due to the development of acute lung injury and ARDS
- Renal failure due to hypotension and capillary bed microthrombus
- Cardiovascular failure as a result of vasodilatation causing hypotension
- Hepatic failure due to microischaemia
- Coagulation failure due to massive overactivation in response to inflammatory mediators
- Central nervous system failure due to hypoperfusion and circulating toxins
- Gut failure due to hypoperfusion and microischaemia

The treatment of sepsis is largely supportive. There is recent evidence to suggest that aggressive resuscitation in the first 6 hours after presentation reduces 28-day mortality. This early goal-directed therapy consists of the administration of fluids and vasopressors with invasive monitoring to keep:

- Mean arterial pressure > 65 mmHg
- Central venous pressure 8–12 mmHg
- Urine output > 0.5ml/kg per hour
- Central venous oxygen saturation > 70%

The subsequent treatment of sepsis includes:

- Fluid therapy to maintain CVP and urine output
- Vasopressors to support blood pressure
- Antibiotics to treat underlying infective cause
- Mechanical ventilation as per ARDS strategies
- Steroids, eg hydrocortisone 100 mg tds for 7 days
- Insulin
- Renal replacement therapy – in the presence of refractory renal failure and metabolic acidosis
- Activated protein C – in the most seriously ill septic patients this has been shown to improve survival (local protocols will apply in all units)

Many patients with sepsis have adrenal depression though there is limited evidence that administration of steroids improves outcome. Intensive glycaemic control, keeping glucose between 4.4 mmol/l and 6.1 mmol/l, has been shown to improve outcome in septic patients.

RENAL REPLACEMENT THERAPY

Renal replacement therapy (RRT) is given in the critical care unit to patients with acute renal failure (ARF). The cause of the ARF is usually sepsis, but is occasionally seen in hypotensive, hypovolaemic patients postoperatively. Acute tubular necrosis causes the kidneys to be unable to excrete waste products and fluid, leading to a uraemic, acidotic, hyperkalaemic, fluid-overloaded patient.

The indications for emergency RRT are:

- Hyperkalaemia not responding to medical treatment
- Resistant and worsening metabolic acidosis when this is due to renal failure alone
- Clinical uraemia (coma, pericarditis)
- Resistant symptoms of fluid overload (pulmonary oedema)

Outside these indications, RRT will usually wait until the light of day.

Broadly speaking, there are two types of RRT employed on the ICU: haemodialysis and haemofiltration. Both rely on the heparinised circulating blood being pumped from the body and passed through a filter with a selectively permeable membrane. In filtration, waste products are squeezed out into a bag, and then volume replaced downstream with a fluid containing known electrolyte concentrations. In dialysis, the filter is bathed in a dialysate, so electrolytes and water can diffuse back across the filter in the opposite way to the waste products.

In general, in the unstable septic patient, haemofiltration is superior as it provides a more instant and controllable means to resolve fluid overload. Also, pump speeds are slower and there are fewer haemodynamic effects (ie hypotension) than are seen with dialysis.

Most units now practise continuous haemofiltration in the septic patient, allowing constant adjustment of fluid, electrolyte and acid/base balance with minimal haemodynamic side-effects.

INOTROPES AND VASOPRESSORS

Many patients on the ICU are hypotensive, and require haemodynamic support with drugs. Inotropes act on the heart to increase contractility and rate, whereas vasopressors cause peripheral and splanchnic (gut bed) vasoconstriction. All patients on these drugs should have a central and arterial line as a minimum.

Commonly used inotropes are:

- Dobutamine – stimulates the heart directly and causes increased contractility. Its use may be limited by the development of significant tachycardia
- Dopexamine – as dobutamine, but may also protect splanchnic circulation

Commonly used vasopressors are:

- Adrenaline/metaraminol (given in boluses in rescue situations)
- Noradrenaline (given as infusion, usually in septic patients)

In the rescue scenario, adrenaline can be given as boluses or an infusion, and will have inotropic and vasopressor properties. None of the above drugs should be commenced on any patient without senior medical input.

SEDATION

Sedation is an important part of intensive care medicine. It is needed to enable critically ill patients requiring ventilation to be intubated and then artificially ventilated. It is also important as it decreases the stress and pain of being in the ICU.

All 'sedation' regimens actually have three aims; namely, anxiolysis, amnesia and analgesia. Most sedative drugs used have properties of the former two, but not analgesia, so a separate, usually opioid, agent is used. All the following drugs are sedative and respiratory depressants, and should not be used without senior advice.

Commonly used sedative drugs:

- Propofol – this is an anaesthetic induction agent which can also be given in infusion. It has a relatively short half-life. It can cause potent vasodilatation, especially in septic patients
- Midazolam – this is a benzodiazepine-type drug which is a potent amnesic

All sedative drugs build in the system over a few days of use, and may require a 'wash-out' period after stopping before the patient fully awakens.

Commonly used analgesics:

- Morphine – given as infusion and titrated to level of pain. Useful especially in postoperative patients. May build up in renal failure. May cause dependency with prolonged use
- Alfentanil – this is a synthetic opioid with a short half-life. It is useful in patients who are likely to require only a short period of ventilation as it does not build up. Also safe in renal failure
- Remifentanyl – this ultra-short-acting synthetic opioid is useful in patients in whom a short but intense period of analgesia is needed, eg for burns dressings

Sedation should always be monitored by a sedation score, such as the one below.

NUTRITION

This area is often poorly dealt with in the critically ill, who are usually malnourished. As patients are often sedated and ventilated, and may have surgical problems, oral feeding is not possible.

- Nasogastric feeding is the most commonly used route in ICU patients. Proprietary feed can be infused up to around 2 litres per day, with a 4-hour 'rest period'. Some patients do not absorb their feed and vomit. In these cases, prokinetic agents such as metoclopramide or erythromycin may be used
- Nasojejunal feeding requires a tube to be placed endoscopically, and is useful in patients with gastric or duodenal pathology
- Total parenteral nutrition should only be used if there is gut failure. It must be given via a central line, and there is a high incidence of line infection

There is now reasonable evidence for the early use of nasogastric feed in the critically ill, and this should be continued to the point where the patient can orally meet their nutritional requirement.

BRAINSTEM DEATH AND ORGAN DONATION

Occasionally, a patient with a catastrophic intracranial event such as a traumatic brain injury or massive subarachnoid haemorrhage will be admitted to the ICU. It is usually clear that recovery is impossible. In this group of patients, brainstem death may occur, with preservation of vital physiological functions. Due to massive increases in intracranial pressure, the brainstem is forced down through the foramen magnum in a process called coning.

Brainstem death must be confirmed by two doctors, fully registered for at least 5 years. Convention dictates that two sets of tests are performed at least 6 hours apart. The time of death is usually taken to be the time of the first set of tests.

Once brainstem death is confirmed, the patient may be considered for organ donation. Following discussion and consent from the next of kin, the regional transplant co-ordinator will be contacted, and they will advise which organs are suitable for retrieval, which tests are needed, and whether any treatment alteration is advised. A retrieval team attends the hospital and retrieves the organs in theatre under anaesthetic. Following this process, the transplant co-ordinator will usually feed back information on organ recipients and their progress. While the process of brainstem testing and donation can be harrowing for staff and relatives, learning the end-results of the process is one of the most gratifying parts of intensive care.

CHAPTER 11

MEDICINE FOR SURGEONS

M O MURPHY AND J GREENWOOD

INTRODUCTION

Many patients admitted to hospital for elective or emergency surgical care have chronic medical conditions which can complicate their management. In addition to dealing with these problems, many postoperative medical complications can occur. This chapter attempts to address many of these, and to provide a guide to how to approach them.

RESPIRATORY PROBLEMS

A request to review a postoperative patient who has become short of breath is a common call to be encountered. On receiving such a request, some simple information may help to prioritise the urgency of review. In general, patients with a respiratory rate of more than 28 breaths per minute, oxygen saturations of less than 90% or cardiovascular compromise require urgent attention. On arrival at the patient's bedside, the initial approach should be **A**irway, **B**reathing and **C**irculation.

- A – are there any signs of airway obstruction, ie stridor? If these are present, seek emergency anaesthetic and senior help
- B – put the patient onto the highest concentration of inspired oxygen you can (probably 15 litres of oxygen via a non-rebreather mask), unless there are any specific contraindications. Assess the respiratory rate and pattern and measure the oxygen saturations. Listen to the chest for air entry, wheezes or crackles
- C – check heart rate and blood pressure

This initial primary survey should allow an initial differential diagnosis to be reached, and initial therapy started. Then request an urgent CXR and check ABG levels if appropriate. Do not delay initial management while waiting for the results of these tests. Careful attention to the patient's previous medical history and usual prescription may give clues to the diagnosis.

POSTOPERATIVE PNEUMONIA

Pneumonia is common in surgical patients, particularly in those with pre-existing chest problems and patients undergoing major abdominal or thoracic surgery. Pain from large incisions may compromise chest expansion and coughing, leading to build up of secretions and basal collapse. Attempts to reduce this can be made by the use of epidural infusions and chest physiotherapy, but despite these measures, pneumonia is still prevalent.

History

Fever, chest pain and cough productive of purulent sputum.

Examination

- Raised respiratory rate
- Decreased oxygen saturations
- Bronchial breathing
- Crackles or decreased air entry over the affected area
- Possible pleural rub

Investigations

- ↑ WCC count and C-reactive protein
- Low oxygen levels on ABG measurement
- There may be consolidation on CXR
- It is essential to send sputum for culture

Treatment

- Oxygen, chest physiotherapy, adequate analgesia and antibiotics
- The first–line antibiotic for hospital-acquired pneumonia varies from Trust to Trust, but most usually is a second- or third-generation cephalosporin or a quinolone (eg ciprofloxacin). Dual therapy, as for severe community-acquired pneumonia, is not generally indicated

PULMONARY OEDEMA

Patients with chronic heart failure and ischaemic heart disease are at risk of pulmonary oedema postoperatively. They are likely to have had their usual diuretic and cardiac medication stopped in the perioperative period, and may have had several litres of intravenous fluid in theatre and recovery.

History

Breathlessness, inability to lie flat and the sensation of drowning.

Examination

- Raised respiratory rate
- Hypoxia
- Frothy secretions from chest and bilateral crackles in lung fields
- Occasionally wheeze may be present

Investigations

- ABG – show hypoxia
- ECG – may show ischaemic changes or a tachyarrhythmia
- CXR – may show bilateral air space shadowing

Treatment

Oxygen, intravenous opioids and intravenous diuretics (eg furosemide 40–80 mg). Pulmonary oedema persisting despite the above is likely to require treatment with intravenous nitrates and possibly respiratory support. Ideally these should be carried out on a coronary care unit under the supervision of a physician. In cases where pulmonary oedema is suspected but by no means clear cut, then there is little harm in giving diuretics, but opioids should be given with caution.

PULMONARY EMBOLUS

Having surgery of any kind and the immobilisation that inevitably follows major surgery puts patients at high risk of thromboembolic disease. Orthopaedic lower limb surgery, gynaecology and urology (lithotomy position), major abdominal procedures and any procedure for malignancy confer additional risk.

PE typically occurs hours to days after surgery. It is important to realise that while the use of prophylactic LMWH has greatly reduced the incidence of PE, it is by no means 100% effective.

A DVT may be clinically apparent and even being treated, but the sudden onset of chest pain and breathlessness should be taken seriously until PE is firmly excluded.

History

Very sudden onset of dyspnoea, with or without pleuritic chest pain. May be symptoms associated with DVT.

Examination

- Increased heart and respiratory rate
- May be hypotensive
- Chest is typically clear

Investigations

- Bloods – usually normal
- ABG – may show hypoxia with a low CO_2
- CXR – typically normal
- The commonest ECG abnormality is sinus tachycardia

Treatment

- Essentially supportive
- Give oxygen and fluid resuscitation if shocked
- Give treatment dose LMWH
- D-dimer estimation is useless in the postoperative patient. Its specificity (reliability at excluding PE if negative) is 98%, but may be falsely negative, especially in high-risk groups. A positive D-dimer is invariable in the immediate postoperative period
- Troponin T is frequently measured in any patient suffering chest pain; this may be positive in PE with no myocardial infarct or ischaemia
- Definitive diagnosis or exclusion of PE is important in deciding long-term treatment. The gold standard investigation is now CT pulmonary angiography in most hospitals, and there are protocols to guide in the request of this test

CHRONIC OBSTRUCTIVE PULMONARY DISEASE AND ASTHMA

While the underlying pathology and chronic management of patients with chronic obstructive pulmonary disease (COPD) and asthma are quite different, the approach to patients suffering an acute exacerbation on the surgical ward is similar. The trigger of an acute attack may be infection, allergic reaction, inadvertent omission of usual treatment or a stress response.

History

Breathless, tight-chested, panicking.

Examination

- Increased heart and respiratory rate, use of accessory muscles, wheeze on chest examination
- Very poor air entry or a silent chest in an asthmatic indicates life-threatening bronchospasm, and immediate senior medical help should be sought

Investigations

- ABG – may show type I or type II respiratory failure (see below). Type II respiratory failure is associated with poor outcome in either group
- CXR – to exclude precipitating factors, eg a pneumothorax

Treatment

Give oxygen, but with caution in the COPD patient, see below. Give nebulised bronchodilators (salbutamol 2.5 mg) at least every 15 minutes and a single dose of steroids, (prednisolone 40 mg by mouth or hydrocortisone 200 mg intravenously, neither is superior). If the patient fails to improve after 30 minutes, seek senior help as the patient may require positive pressure ventilation or intubation.

Patients with more severe COPD may develop chronic hypercapnia. Their respiratory centres become used to the higher carbon dioxide levels, and their stimulus to breathe becomes chronic hypoxia. If this is corrected with the use of too much oxygen, then they hypoventilate, retain carbon dioxide and become acidotic. As such, patients with COPD should be given oxygen with great caution. It should only ever be given in a controlled fashion at a known concentration (ie via a Venturi mask). Oxygen saturations of 90–92% in these patients are entirely satisfactory and should not be exceeded. If patients do require higher concentrations of oxygen for any reason, regular blood gas measurements should be done.

PRIMARY HYPERVENTILATION

Hyperventilation in surgical patients may occur for many reasons, especially pain. However in a small number of tachypnoeic patients no pathological cause may be apparent and may be psychological in origin. This conclusion should only be reached after careful exclusion of other conditions.

History

Breathlessness, sensation of choking, lightheadedness, tingling of fingertips and spasm of small muscles of hands.

Examination

Most likely none, apart from raised respiratory rate.

Investigations

ABG show raised oxygen and low carbon dioxide.

Treatment

Reassurance and re-breathing into paper bag if necessary.

CARDIOVASCULAR PROBLEMS

Cardiovascular problems in the surgical patient can range from a minor angina attack to catastrophic hypotension and myocardial infarction. Patients with otherwise stable ischaemic heart disease or arrhythmia are subjected to abnormal stresses which may precipitate attacks, and often have some or all of their normal medication stopped in the perioperative period.

CHEST PAIN

This is probably the most common call received.

History

It is important to determine first off whether or not the patient has a history of ischaemic heart disease. The patient will usually be able to tell you whether this is an angina attack, or if it feels different or worse.

Examination

- Check temperature, pulse, BP
- Full cardiac and respiratory examination

Investigations

- The most important initial step is to obtain a 12-lead ECG. ST segment elevation of more than 2 mm in two adjacent chest leads or 1 mm in adjacent limb leads, or new left bundle branch block is indicative of acute myocardial infarction

- FBC – anaemia
- U&E – renal failure, K$^+$ imbalance
- Troponin T after 12 hours
- BM

Treatment

Initial management is to give oxygen and nitrates. Again, the patient is likely to have a glyceryl trinitrate (GTN) spray. If this fails to settle, or a 12-lead ECG shows any signs of ischaemia (ST segment depression, new T wave inversion), then repeated doses of GTN or opioids may be needed.

Rarely, an episode of severe chest pain in a surgical patient represents acute coronary syndrome. This includes ST elevation myocardial infarction (STEMI), non-ST elevation MI (NSTEMI) and unstable angina. Clearly the gold-standard treatment, namely thrombolysis, is inappropriate in postoperative patients or those with unstable surgical problems.

Initial management should be oxygen, opioids and nitrates, then seek urgent senior medical help. If there are no ST segment changes, but prolonged pain, then the management is the same, but a troponin T level should be checked 12 hours after the onset of pain. If raised, then specialist cardiology review is required. Postoperative myocardial infarction is associated with high mortality and significant rate of reinfarction (Table 11.1).

It is important to compare ECGs taken during an acute episode with older ECGs from the case notes, as abnormalities may be longstanding and thus not require acute management.

Table 11.1 Post-myocardial infarction risk of reinfarction perioperatively

< 3 weeks	80%
3 weeks – 3 months	20–30%
3–6 months	5–15%
> 6 months	1–4%
Perioperative MI mortality	50%
Baseline perioperative MI rate is 0.2% of which half are silent and most are on the third postoperative day	

ATRIAL FIBRILLATION AND ARRHYTHMIAS

Atrial fibrillation is a normal finding in those over 80. However, if left untreated, atrial fibrillation with a fast ventricular response can cause ischaemia and pulmonary oedema, and predisposes to systemic embolisation of thrombus. In surgical patients the commonest causes of fast atrial fibrillation are abnormal fluid balance, electrolyte disturbance, pain and lack of normal medication.

History

It is important to determine whether a patient you are called to see with fast atrial fibrillation on the ward has pre-existing atrial fibrillation, and whether the rate is compromising blood pressure.

Treatment

If the blood pressure is compromised, use the following approach:

- Give a fluid bolus, eg 250 ml succinylated gelatin (Gelofusine)
- Seek urgent senior help
- Consider cardioversion. Initially this should be by giving a bolus of amiodarone 300 mg

If the blood pressure is not compromised, then the following steps should be taken:

- Assess fluid balance and if underfilled then give a gentle fluid bolus
- Check electrolytes in particular K^+, Mg^{2+}, Ca^{2+} and correct as indicated
- If pre-existing atrial fibrillation and medication missed, give digoxin or amiodarone orally or intravenously

Most patients will revert to sinus rhythm or slow their ventricular response with these simple measures.

There are numerous causes of hypotension in the surgical patient, many of which are dealt with elsewhere, but they can be divided into three broad categories:

- Hypovolaemia
- Decreased vascular resistance
- Cardiac insufficiency

The process of identifying the cause of the fall in blood pressure is largely one of exclusion. In the surgical patient, hypovolaemia is generally due to haemorrhage or excessive fluid loss from other routes (ooze, drains), not being matched by fluid input, either orally or intravenously. Relative intravascular volume depletion is manifested by hypotension and a decrease in urine output.

Decreased vascular resistance occurs in surgical patients for many reasons, but the most serious of these is sepsis (see Chapter 10). The other major cause of hypotension is drugs. Patients with medical co-morbidity will invariably be prescribed one or more drugs which have a direct effect on vascular tone and/or cardiac output. In a relatively fluid-depleted patient who has not received these medications for a day or two, the effects of readministration can be pronounced and dramatic. Many analgesics, especially opioids, also cause hypotension. When faced with a hypotensive patient, a reasonable starting point is to give a fluid challenge (suggest 250–500 ml Gelofusine) while assessing for other causes. It is unlikely that this will cause significant pulmonary oedema if the patient is normovolaemic. Basic investigations to rule out bleeding or sepsis can be performed and the drug chart reviewed. If the blood pressure does not improve with simple measures, seek senior help.

Many patients undergoing elective or emergency surgery have cardiac insufficiency and this may be noted in their past medical history or unmasked by their current admission. Ischaemic heart disease puts patients at risk of a perioperative infarct, which in many cases is silent. Valvular heart disease and chronic ventricular dysfunction can also cause cardiac function to be impaired. While overall function may be adequate to cope with everyday activity, the heart struggles to adjust to the increased demands of surgery or the postoperative period.

HYPERTENSION

Many patients with multiple medical problems have chronic hypertension. The presence of significant hypertension in these patients in a surgical setting is likely to represent omission of usual medications combined with stress and pain. Unless the patient has acute malignant hypertension with encephalopathy and papilloedema, there are no indications for the use of sublingual or intravenous agents to lower the blood pressure. In most cases, re-establishment on the usual drug regimen will be sufficient. Patients with hypertension which is untreated can usually be referred to a physician or their general practitioner for management of this as an outpatient.

THE UNCONSCIOUS PATIENT

It is not uncommon to be asked to see a patient on the ward who has become unconscious or cannot be woken. This is a distinct group from those presenting to A&E (dealt with in Chapter 7). As always, the approach to them should be:

- **A** – ensure that they have a patent airway. If not, an oropharyngeal or a nasopharyngeal airway should be inserted
- **B** – are they breathing? If they are, is the rate and pattern normal? Check pulse oximetry
- **C** – do they have a pulse and if so is it normal in rate and rhythm? What is the blood pressure and capillary refill?
- Are they rousable to voice or pain? Quickly estimate the GCS (see Table 7.1, page 264). Check the pupils are reactive to light
- Any signs of injury, bleeding, etc
- Following this quick assessment, a diagnosis can be looked for and a more detailed examination be carried out

Intracranial events are a rare cause of falling GCS in surgical patients. Examination often reveals unequal pupils, a unilateral weakness and abnormal plantar responses uni- or bilaterally. A history of head injury or alcohol excess may mean subdural bleed.

A history of atrial fibrillation, ischaemic heart disease or hypertension may mean cerebral infarct. Be aware of the patient on warfarin or heparin and these must be stopped immediately and reversed if needed. CT brain scan must be carried out within 24 hours if the GCS is normal but there is focal neurology, and immediately if there is depression of the GCS with focal neurology.

It is important to check the drug chart, particularly for recently administered medication as many drugs used in postoperative patients depress the CNS. Opioid analgesics directly depress the consciousness level and also respiratory drive, especially in elderly or underweight patients, and in those with renal failure. If the patient is unarousable and their respiration is depressed, give naloxone (200–400 μg) to reverse the opioid. Benzodiazepines are used as anxiolytics and sedatives in day-case and endoscopic procedures. These may contribute to consciousness level depression. If you suspect this, seek urgent senior help. Many drugs used in postoperative nausea control are mildly sedative (cyclizine, metoclopramide).

If the patient has COPD and is on a high concentration of inspired oxygen, immediately remove or decrease the oxygen flow and check arterial blood gases.

Diabetic patients are usually given iv insulin if having major surgery. They also do not eat very much around this time. All unconscious patients, especially those with diabetes, should have a blood glucose level checked, and glucose should be given if this is low (<2.5 mmol/l). Local guidelines may require 50% glucose solution to be administered via a central line only due to the venocorrosive effects. However, no one ever dies of thrombophlebitis, so glucose administration must not be omitted or delayed due to this guidance.

THE CONFUSED PATIENT

Many patients become confused while in hospital. This is particularly true in elderly patients. Patients with pre-existing dementia can become very disorientated simply by moving to a different environment. Causes of confusion that should be considered and either excluded or treated include:

- Drugs (analgesics, sedatives, antiemetics, omission of normal medications)
- Dehydration
- Pain
- Infection (urinary tract, chest, skin)
- Constipation
- Cerebral event
- Hypoxia
- Renal failure
- Hypoglycaemia

THE FITTING PATIENT

Seizures are an uncommon occurrence in surgical patients outside neurosurgical wards. If associated with head injury, an urgent CT brain is indicated once the seizures are under control. Seizures de novo also require investigation, and referral to a physician is indicated.

The two most likely scenarios are the known epileptic patient who has missed doses of medication, or who fits due to the surgical insult, and the withdrawing substance misuser. Whatever the underlying cause, the approach to the fitting patient is the same:

- Assess (as always) **A B C**
- Establish intravenous access
- Give diazepam emulsion (Diazemuls) 2.5- to 5-mg boluses iv or rectally, up to a maximum of 30 mg, until the seizures stop
- If the seizures do not terminate it is likely they will require further anticonvulsants

Known epileptics should be re-established on their usual regimen as soon as possible after surgery. Substance withdrawal can be treated with chlordiazepoxide and other substitutes (see Alcohol withdrawal, page 368). The use of intravenous anticonvulsants such as phenytoin should only be following senior medical input.

RENAL FAILURE (See Chapter 10)

Renal failure is commonly seen in surgical patients. Occasionally a patient with chronic failure on dialysis will require elective or emergency surgery. In this situation, management should be in close conjunction with the local renal centre who will provide support and advice, and a plan for pre- and postoperative RRT (renal replacement therapy). RRT may take the form of haemofiltration, formal haemodialysis, peritoneal dialysis or transplantation. In acute renal failure (ARF), only the first two are used.

The most likely scenario, however, is the patient with normal or mildly impaired renal function who has acute renal failure (ARF), either pre-operatively as a consequence of their underlying pathology, or post-operatively as a result of hypovolaemia or sepsis.

Renal failure can be broadly divided into three types:

- **Prerenal** – where the insult is related to a decreased fluid delivery to the kidney, ie hypovolaemia of any cause. In a surgical patient this is haemorrhage, sepsis or inadequate fluid balance, and is by far the commonest class of renal failure seen. Serum urea may be disproportionately raised compared to creatinine
- **Intrinsic to the kidney** – where the insult is direct to the renal parenchyma, eg glomerulonephritis. In a surgical patient this is rare, but may be a manifestation of sepsis
- **Postrenal** – due to obstruction of the renal outflow, eg a blocked catheter or carcinoma of bladder obstructing the ureter. This is seen mostly in urology patients, but any abdominal pathology which may invade or involve the bladder or ureters may cause this

History

The most likely initially noted abnormality will be a rising urea and creatinine. It is important to compare the results to any old results from the case notes to assess whether there is chronic renal impairment. It is also important to monitor urine output, and a fall in this may point to hypovolaemia. Severe ARF causes acute tubular necrosis, with persistent hyperkalaemia and metabolic acidosis.

Investigations

In suspected or confirmed ARF, check the following, and monitor at least 6 hourly in the acute phase, and daily until returned to normal:

- Serum potassium. If levels > 6 mmol/l this needs urgent treatment.
- Serum urea. Clinical signs of uraemia include confusion, twitching, pericardial rub
- Serum creatinine
- ABG
- De novo ARF requires a renal ultrasound scan to rule out obstruction and assess the kidney size. Small scarred kidneys are characteristic of long-standing pathology.

Treatment

- If potassium > 7 mmol/l there is imminent risk of cardiac arrhythmia. Give calcium gluconate 10%, 10 ml iv bolus. This is cardioprotective
- Hyperkalaemia is treated with Actrapid insulin/Humulin S 15 units, given in 50 ml dextrose 50% over 15 minutes. Repeated doses can be given until potassium < 6 mmol/l
- If there is a metabolic acidosis, ie pH < 7.35, pCO_2 < 4.5 kPa, bicarbonate < 20 mmol/l, seek senior help as the patient is likely to require RRT
- Assess fluid balance clinically and with CVP measurement
- If dry, hypotensive or oliguric, give fluid challenge of Gelofusine 500 ml. If urine output picks up with this, provide greater fluid input
- If the urine output is poor **DO NOT** give diuretics unless adequate assessment of fluid balance has been made and senior help has been sought. You could make things worse

---

INDICATIONS FOR URGENT DIALYSIS

- Resistant hyperkalaemia despite repeated dextrose/insulin therapy
- Worsening metabolic acidosis
- Resistant fluid overload causing pulmonary oedema
- Gross clinical uraemia, ie coma or pericarditis

ALCOHOL WITHDRAWAL

Classic features are sweating, tremors and agitation after 1–3 days abstinence. The only feature may be confusion but severe cases may result in fits. In withdrawing patients, give:

- Chlordiazepoxide 20 mg qds and as required as a decreasing regimen. Many pharmacy departments produce proformas for prescribing decreasing dose regimens
- Pabrinex (I and II) three times daily intravenously for the first 3 days to prevent Wernicke's encephalopathy

ANAPHYLAXIS

This is a profound allergic reaction, usually to a drug, especially antibiotics, but occasionally to latex, Elastoplast or iodine to name but a few. Features are hypotension, flushing, wheezing, stridor, facial oedema and skin rashes.

Treatment

Give chlorphenamine 10 mg iv, hydrocortisone 200 mg iv, and if this does not settle things or there is shock or facial swelling, give adrenaline 1:1000, 1mg **intramuscularly**.

- **Seek immediate senior help**

BLOOD TRANSFUSION

Usually this is needed when there has been surgical blood loss. Generally, transfusion is not required unless the haemoglobin is less than 80 g/l, except if there is active haemorrhage. Patients **do not** require diuretics with blood transfusions unless they are known to have severe left ventricular failure or renal failure causing fluid retention.

DEEP VEIN THROMBOSIS

RISK FACTORS

- Any prolonged surgical procedure, especially orthopaedic, gynaecology and abdominal
- Malignancy of any site
- Previous DVT
- Prolonged immobility
- Smoking
- Use of hormone replacement or oral contraceptive medications
- Dehydration

History

- Pain, warmth and swelling of affected leg

Examination

- Obvious unilateral leg swelling, calf tenderness, redness and warmth

Investigations

The test of choice is a Doppler leg vein ultrasound. However some departments will still insist on a venogram. If the history and examination are highly suggestive of DVT but the test is negative, then a repeat scan 1 week later is indicated. D-Dimer estimation in the postoperative patient is a waste of time.

Treatment

- An above-knee DVT should be treated with anticoagulation for 6 months

DIABETES MELLITUS

Patients with diabetes who are having surgery need their blood glucose closely controlled around the time of operation. The anaesthetist will usually advise when this is to be started, and will be a sliding scale insulin infusion or a GKI protocol depending on local preference. Generally, this should be continued until the patient is eating and drinking normally in the postoperative period, at which point the patient's usual diabetic medication can be restarted.

Do not be tempted or bullied into giving small boluses of short-acting insulin to the diabetic patient whose blood sugar is slightly high. This will cause the glycaemic control to go haywire and will make it impossible to follow trends and adjust long-term treatment accordingly.

Mildly abnormal LFT in hospital inpatients is common. Usually the cause is drugs (antibiotics) or sepsis, and the abnormality corrects once the precipitant is removed. Many patients who come in to hospital are already malnourished, often as a result of the process for which they are admitted. Then, we starve them for surgery, keep them nil by mouth postoperatively, make them vomit and feed them unappetising hospital food. Careful attention to nutrition is important. The dietetics department can advise on supplements. Patients commencing nasogastric or jejunal feed or total parenteral nutrition require close monitoring of electrolytes and correction of abnormalities to prevent the re-feeding syndrome.

INDEX